MAYO CLINIC

Book of
HOME
REMEDIES

SECOND EDITION

MAYO CLINIC PRESS

Published by Mayo Clnic Press

© 2017 Mayo Foundation for Medical Education and Research (MFMER)

For bulk sales to employers, member groups and health-related companies, write Mayo Clinic, 200 First St. SW, Rochester, MN 55905, call 800-430-9699, or email *SpecialSalesMayoBooks@mayo.edu*.

ISBN 13: 978-1-893005-68-6

Printed in the USA

Mayo Clinic

MEDICAL EDITORS
Cindy A. Kermott, M.D., M.P.H.
Martha P. Millman, M.D., M.P.H.

EDITORIAL DIRECTOR
Paula M. Marlow Limbeck

SENIOR EDITOR
Karen R. Wallevand

MANAGING EDITOR
Jennifer L. Jacobson

PRODUCT MANAGER
Christopher C. Frye

ILLUSTRATION, PHOTOGRAPHY AND PRODUCTION
Kent Mc Daniel, Matthew C. Meyer, Gunnar T. Soroos, Malgorzata (Gosha) B. Weivoda

EDITORIAL RESEARCH
Abbie Y. Brown, Deirdre A. Herman, Erika A. Riggin

PROOFREADING
Miranda M. Attlesey, Alison K. Baker, Julie M. Maas

INDEXING
Steve Rath

ADMINISTRATIVE ASSISTANT
Terri L. Zanto Strausbauch

CONTRIBUTORS
Daniel A. Assad, D.D.S., Sophie J. Bakri, M.D., Keith A. Bengtson, M.D., Christopher (Chris) L. Boswell, M.D., Jeffrey S. Brault, D.O., Petra M. Casey, M.D., Bart L. Clarke, M.D., David W. Claypool, M.D., Martin G. Ellman, D.P.M., Floranne C. Ernste, M.D., Kevin C. Fleming, M.D., Amy E. Foxx-Orenstein, D.O., Matthew T. Gettman, M.D., Karthik Ghosh, M.D., Cynthia A. Hogan, Ph.D., W. Michael Hooten, M.D., Robert M. Jacobson, M.D., Amer N. Kalaaji, M.D., Mary J. Kasten, M.D., Frank P. Kennedy, M.D., Stephen L. Kopecky, M.D., Lois E. Krahn, M.D., Esther H. Krych, M.D., Devyani Lal, M.D., James T. Li, M.D., Ph.D., Sharon E. Libi, M.D., Kevin G. Moder, M.D., Robin G. Molella, M.D., M.P.H., Brian A. Neff, M.D., Eric J. Olson, M.D., David E. Patterson, M.D., Carrie (Beth) E. Robertson, M.D., Teresa A. Rummans, M.D., Priya Sampathkumar, M.D., Nicole P. Sandhu, M.D., Ph.D., James M. Steckelberg, M.D., Sandra J. Taler, M.D., Carmen M. Terzic, M.D., Ph.D., Jacqueline M. Thielen, M.D., Gerald W. Volcheck, M.D., Debra A. Zillmer, M.D.

Table of contents

Table of contents continued

Introduction

Today, greater responsibility has been placed on you as an individual to stay healthy and prevent illness. This has been triggered, in no small part, by the rising costs of health care and by growing concern over public health issues as diverse as obesity, diabetes, influenza and food safety.

Of course, things happen that you may have little control over — even after taking precautions, you may still catch colds, sprain ankles, have allergic reactions or develop high blood pressure. This book can show you how to minimize your risks of disease and injury. And in the event that something should happen, it shows necessary steps to take to help treat the condition until it's resolved or until you're able to see your doctor.

How the book is organized

Considering the broad spectrum of health issues included in this book, the topics are arranged alphabetically. Each topic is introduced in a summary that may include signs and symptoms, causes, and possible outcomes.

Accompanying each topic is a "Home remedies" segment that describes simple actions you can take to help prevent, treat or manage the condition, whether it's straightforward advice on diet and exercise, change in behavior, or a supplement to help relieve signs and symptoms.

The "Medical help" segment with each topic identifies serious signs and symptoms and advises you on when to contact a doctor or other health care provider and what kind of treatment you might expect.

The *Mayo Clinic Book of Home Remedies* is based on the premise that there are many things you can do at home to stay healthy, relieve symptoms, improve emotional health, feel invigorated and enjoy a higher quality of life. We hope that it provides you with an important resource in achieving this complete approach to good health.

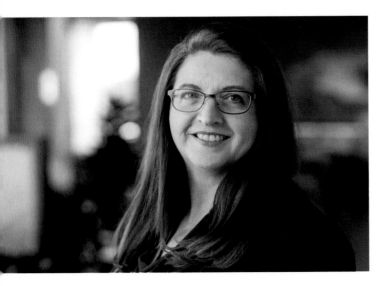

Cindy A. Kermott, M.D., M.P.H.
Medical editor, *Mayo Clinic Book of Home Remedies*, Second Edition, specialist in the Executive Health Program and medical director of Preventive Services Clinic, Mayo Clinic, Rochester, Minnesota.

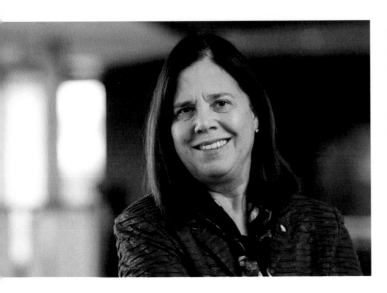

Martha P. Millman, M.D., M.P.H.
Medical editor, *Mayo Clinic Book of Home Remedies*, Second Edition, and emeritus physician with career expertise in preventive medicine, hyperbaric medicine and wound care, Mayo Clinic, Rochester, Minnesota.

Medical supplies for your home

When an accident or health problem occurs, it's nice to have basic supplies on hand to treat the condition. That's why you want to have a medical supply kit ready for use — whether it's an actual first-aid kit or just your bathroom cabinet stocked with a variety of helpful items.

It's best to store medical supplies in a place that's easily accessible to adults but out of the reach of children. Remember to replace items after their use to make sure the kit is always complete. And check your supplies yearly for outdated items that may need replacing. Check expiration dates on medications twice yearly.

Here are key items that you should have on hand if you want to be prepared for accidents and common illnesses:

- **For general care.** Sharp scissors, tweezers, cotton balls, cotton-tipped swabs, tissues, soap, cleansing pads or instant hand sanitizer, plastic bags, safety pins, latex or synthetic gloves for use if blood or body fluids are present, anti-diarrheal drugs, and a medicine cup or spoon.
- **For cuts.** Bandages of various sizes, gauze, paper or cloth tape, antiseptic solution to clean wounds, and antibacterial ointment to prevent infection.
- **For burns.** Cold packs, gauze, burn spray and antiseptic cream.
- **For aches, pain and fever.** Thermometer, aspirin (for adults only), other pain-relieving drugs such as ibuprofen (Advil, Motrin IB, others), and acetaminophen (Tylenol, others).
- **For eye injuries.** Eyewash, such as saline solution, eyewash cup, eye patches and goggles.
- **For sprains, strains and fractures.** Cold packs, elastic wraps for wrapping injuries, finger splints and a triangular bandage for making an arm sling.
- **For insect bites and stings.** Cold packs to help reduce pain and swelling. Topical cream containing hydrocortisone (0.5 or 1 percent), calamine lotion, or baking soda (combine baking soda with water to form a paste) to apply until symptoms subside. Antihistamines (Benadryl, Chlor-Trimeton, others) may help relieve itching. For individuals allergic to insect stings, include a kit with a syringe containing epinephrine (adrenaline). Your doctor can prescribe one. Check the expiration date regularly.
- **For ingestion of poisons.** Keep the number of the U.S. Poison Help line (800-222-1222) in your medicine kit or programmed into your phone.

Emergency items

Here are additional items you may want to have on hand in case of an emergency at home or while traveling:

- Cellphone and charger that uses the accessory plug in your car's dash
- Emergency phone numbers, including contact information for your family doctor and pediatrician, local emergency services, emergency road service providers and poison control center
- Completed authorization to disclose protected health information (consent form) for each family member
- Medical history forms for each family member
- Small, waterproof flashlight and extra batteries
- Candles and matches and an extra set of warm clothing for cold climates
- Sunscreen
- Mylar emergency blanket
- First-aid instruction manual

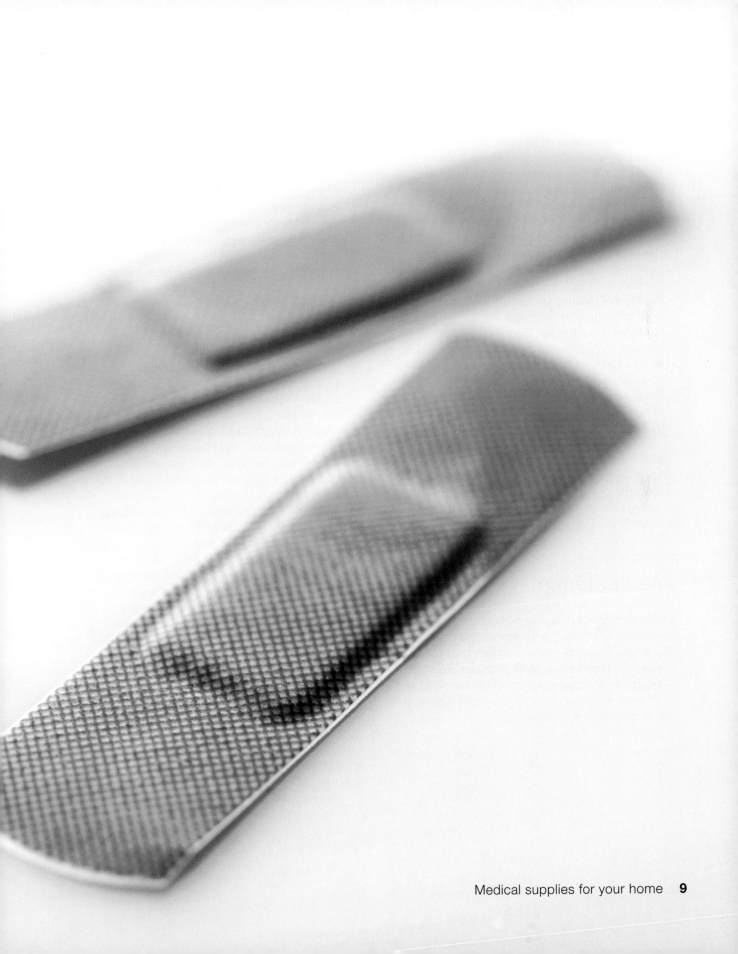

Acne

Acne occurs when the tiny openings in your skin from which hair grows (hair follicles) become plugged with oil and dead skin cells. The plugged follicles may produce:

- **Comedones (blackheads and whiteheads).** Comedones that occur at the skin surface are called blackheads due to their dark appearance. Comedones that are closed and just below the skin surface are called whiteheads.
- **Papules.** Papules are small, red and tender bumps that signal inflammation or infection in the hair follicles.
- **Pustules.** Pustules are red and tender bumps with white pus at their tips.
- **Nodules.** Nodules are large, solid painful lumps beneath the surface of the skin. They are the result of a buildup of secretions deep within the hair follicles.
- **Cysts.** These painful, pus-filled lumps beneath the surface of the skin are boil-like infections that can cause scars.

A number of factors — including hormones, bacteria, certain medications and heredity — play a role in the development of acne. Though acne is most common in teenagers, people of all ages can get acne.

Medical help

Persistent pimples, inflamed cysts or scarring may need medical attention and treatment with prescription drugs. Proper evaluation and treatment can prevent the physical and psychological scarring of acne. In rare cases, a sudden onset of severe acne in an older adult may signal an underlying disease requiring medical attention.

Home remedies

To reduce or prevent acne:

- *Be careful what you put on your face.* Avoid oily or greasy cosmetics or hairstyling products or acne coverups. Use products labeled water-based or noncomedogenic.
- *Keep your face clean.* Wash problem areas daily with a gentle cleanser that gently dries your skin. Products such as facial scrubs, astringents and masks generally aren't recommended because they tend to irritate skin, which can worsen acne.
- *Watch what touches your face.* Keep your hair clean and off your face. Avoid resting your hands or objects, such as telephone receivers, on your face. Tight hats also can pose a problem, especially if you sweat. Sweat and dirt can contribute to acne.
- *Care for yourself.* Consider whether lack of sleep or stress or both cause your acne to flare. Try to get enough sleep and manage stress.
- *Don't pick or squeeze blemishes.* Doing so can lead to infection or scarring.
- *Try over-the-counter products.* Look for acne lotions that contain benzoyl peroxide or salicylic acid as the active ingredient to help dry excess oil and promote peeling of dead skin cells.
- *Tea tree oil.* Some studies suggest that gels containing 5 percent tea tree oil are as effective as lotions containing 5 percent benzoyl peroxide, although tea tree oil might work more slowly. There's some concern that topical products containing tea tree oil might cause breast development in young boys. Don't use tea tree oil if you have acne rosacea because it can worsen symptoms.
- *Zinc supplements.* The mineral zinc plays a role in wound healing and reduces inflammation, which may help improve acne.
- *Glycolic acid.* A natural acid found in sugar cane, glycolic acid applied to your skin helps remove dead skin cells and unclog pores.

Airplane ear

The medical name for airplane ear is ear barotrauma, or barotitis media. It refers to the stress exerted on your eardrum, eustachian tube and other ear structures when air pressure in your middle ear and air pressure in the environment are out of balance.

You may experience airplane ear at the beginning of a flight when the airplane is climbing and at the end of a flight when the airplane is descending. These rapid changes in altitude cause air pressure in the environment to also change rapidly. The air pressure in the middle ear does not adjust quickly enough.

Signs and symptoms may include pain in one ear, slight hearing loss or a stuffy feeling in both ears. This is caused by your eardrum bulging outward or retracting inward as a result of the change in pressure.

Ear barotrauma is also a common problem with scuba diving when water pressure on the outside of the ear becomes greater than air pressure in the middle ear.

Any condition that can interfere with the normal function of the middle ear can increase the risk of airplane ear. This would include a stuffy nose, an allergy, a cold or a throat infection. Not all colds require a change in travel plans. However, a severe cold or an ear infection may be reason to change or delay a flight.

Medical help

Usually, you can do things on your own to treat airplane ear. If discomfort, fullness or muffled hearing lasts more than a few hours or if you experience any severe signs or symptoms, call your doctor.

Home remedies

To prevent or reduce airplane ear:

- *Use a decongestant.* Take a decongestant about 30 minutes to an hour before takeoff and 30 minutes to an hour before landing. This may prevent blockage of your eustachian tube. If you have heart disease, a heart rhythm disorder or high blood pressure or if you've experienced possible medication interactions, avoid taking an oral decongestant.
- *During the flight, suck on candy or chew gum.* This encourages swallowing, which helps open your eustachian tube.
- *Don't sleep during ascents and descents.* If you're awake during ascents and descents, you can do the necessary self-care techniques when you feel pressure on your ears.
- *Try the Valsalva maneuver to unplug your ears.* Gently blow, as if blowing your nose, while pinching your nostrils and keeping your mouth closed. If you can swallow at the same time, it's more helpful. Repeat several times to equalize the pressure between your ears and the airplane cabin.
- *Look for specially designed filtered earplugs.* Theses earplugs slowly equalize the pressure against your eardrum during ascents and descents. You can purchase these at drugstores, airport gift shops or your local hearing clinic.
- *Give infants and children fluid.* Drinking fluids during ascent and descent encourages swallowing. Give the child a bottle or pacifier to encourage swallowing. Decongestants should not be used in infants or young children.

Allergies

An allergy is an overreaction by your immune system to an otherwise harmless substance, such as pollen or pet dander.

Contact with this substance — called an allergen — triggers the production of antibodies to fight the invader. The antibodies, in turn, cause immune cells in the lining of your eyes and airways to release inflammatory substances, including histamine.

When these chemicals are released, they produce the familiar signs and symptoms of allergy: itchy, red and swollen eyes; stuffy nose; frequent sneezing; cough; and hives or bumps on the skin.

Many people mistake allergies for colds, but signs and symptoms of these two conditions are different (see page 13). A cold generally goes away in a few days, whereas an allergy often persists for a longer time.

Types

Substances found outdoors and indoors can cause allergic reactions.

The most common allergens are inhaled:

- **Pollen.** Spring, summer and fall are the pollen-producing seasons in many climates, when you're more exposed to airborne particles from trees, grasses and weeds.
- **Dust mites.** House dust harbors many allergens, including pollen and molds. But the main allergy trigger is the dust mite. Thousands of these microscopic insects are in a pinch of house dust. House dust can cause year-round allergy symptoms.
- **Pet dander.** Dogs and especially cats are the most common animals to cause allergic reactions. The animal's dander (skin flakes), saliva, urine and sometimes hair are the main culprits.

- **Molds.** Many people are sensitive to airborne mold spores. Outdoor molds produce spores mostly in the summer and early fall in northern climates and year-round in subtropical and tropical climates. Indoor molds shed spores all year long. People also may develop allergies to certain foods, insect stings, medications and latex, or other things you touch.

Hay fever (allergic rhinitis)

Signs and symptoms generally include a stuffy or runny nose, frequent sneezing, and itchy eyes, nose, throat or mouth. Hay fever may also be accompanied by a cough. Seasonal hay fever triggers include:

- Tree pollen, common in spring
- Grass pollen, common in the late spring and summer
- Weed pollen, most common in the fall
- Spores from fungi and molds, which can be worse during warm-weather months

Medical help

See your doctor if you find your signs and symptoms aren't easily controlled by these steps. A number of prescription medications are available that can lessen or prevent your concerns.

An allergy versus a cold

If you tend to get "colds" that develop suddenly and occur at about the same time every year, it's possible that you actually have a seasonal allergy.

Although colds and seasonal allergies may share some of the same symptoms, they are very different conditions. Common colds are caused by viruses, while seasonal allergies are immune system responses that are triggered by exposure to an allergen.

Treating colds may include rest, pain relievers and over-the-counter cold remedies, such as decongestants. Treating allergies may include taking over-the-counter or prescription antihistamines, nasal steroid sprays, and decongestants, and avoiding or reducing exposure to the allergens where possible.

Is it a cold or an allergy?

Symptom	Cold	Allergy
Cough	Usually	Sometimes
General aches and pains	Sometimes	Never
Fatigue	Sometimes	Sometimes
Itchy eyes	Rarely	Usually
Sneezing	Usually	Usually
Sore throat	Usually	Sometimes
Runny nose	Usually	Usually
Stuffy nose	Usually	Usually
Fever	Rarely	Never

Based on National Institute of Allergy and Infectious Diseases 2014

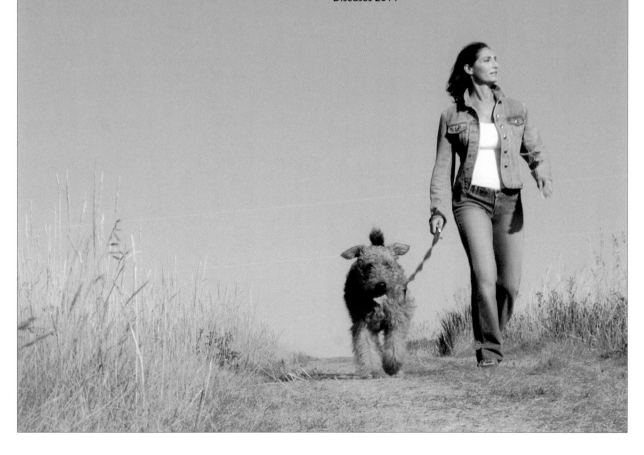

Home remedies

The best approach for managing allergies is to know and avoid your allergy triggers.

Pollen

- *Rinse out your sinuses.* Sinus congestion and hay fever symptoms often improve with nasal lavage — rinsing out the sinuses with a saline solution. You can use a neti pot, a specially designed bulb syringe or nasal bottle irrigation to flush out thickened mucus and irritants from your nose. See page 151.
- *Don't hang laundry outside.* Pollen can stick to the laundry. Also shower and change clothes upon entering your home after outdoor exposure.
- *Close windows and doors during pollen season.* Use an air conditioner with a good filter.
- *Use an allergy-grade filter.* Look for a high-efficiency particulate air (HEPA) filter for your ventilation and heating system. Change filters monthly.
- *Wear a pollen mask.* Use it outdoors for yardwork, or when you're around known triggers.

Dust or mold

- *Limit your exposure.* To prevent dust from building up, clean your home at least once a week. Wear a mask while cleaning, or have someone else clean for you.
- *Encase mattresses and pillows.* Place them in dustproof or allergen-blocking covers. Wash your bedding and pillowcases in hot water on a weekly basis.
- *Redecorate your house.* Consider replacing upholstered furniture with leather or vinyl, and carpeting with wood, vinyl or tile (particularly in the bedroom).
- *Maintain indoor humidity between 30 and 50 percent.* Use kitchen and bathroom exhaust fans and a dehumidifier in the basement.
- *Clean humidifiers and dehumidifiers often.* Thorough cleaning helps prevent mold and bacterial growth in the appliances.
- *Change furnace filters monthly.* Also consider installing a high-efficiency particulate air (HEPA) filter in your heating system.

Pets

- *Be selective about your pets.* Avoid pets with fur or feathers, or look into hypoallergenic breeds.
- *Keep pets out of the bedroom.* If you choose to keep a furry pet, keep it out of the bedroom and in an area of the home that's easily cleaned.
- *Bathe pets weekly.* Using wipes that are specially designed to reduce dander also may help.

Arthritis

Arthritis is one of the most common medical conditions in the United States. There are more than 100 different types of arthritis, which have varying causes, signs and symptoms, and treatments. The most common types of arthritis are osteoarthritis and rheumatoid arthritis.

Osteoarthritis

Osteoarthritis is often associated with wear and tear on one or more of your joints, causing the cartilage to degenerate in your spine, hands, hips or knees. Obesity, aging, injury or genetics can increase your risk. Osteoarthritis is most often seen in people older than age 50. The signs and symptoms include:

- Pain in a joint after use
- Swelling and loss of flexibility in a joint
- Bony lumps at finger joints
- Aching

While the disease doesn't go away, the pain and other signs and symptoms may come and go.

Rheumatoid arthritis

Rheumatoid arthritis is a form of inflammatory arthritis. It most often develops in middle age, but can occur in any age group. The cause is unknown, but it's an autoimmune disease, meaning that your immune system triggers inflammation in the lining of your joints and in other areas. Signs and symptoms of rheumatoid arthritis include:

- Swelling in one or more joints
- Prolonged early-morning stiffness
- Recurring pain or tenderness in any joint
- Inability to move a joint normally
- Obvious redness and warmth in a joint

Medical help

If you have swelling or stiffness in your joints that lasts for more than two weeks, make an appointment with your doctor.

Rub it in

Topical painkillers come as gels, creams, lotions or patches that are applied directly to the skin over your aching joints. Three types that you can purchase without a prescription include:

- *Hot or cold rubs.* Doctors call these products counterirritants because they contain ingredients that irritate your skin. Ingredients such as menthol, oil of wintergreen or eucalyptus oil produce a sensation of hot or cold that distracts you from your arthritis pain, giving you temporary pain relief. Examples include Biofreeze, Flexall and Icy Hot.
- *Aspirin-like pain rubs.* Topical analgesics contain salicylates, the same ingredients that give aspirin its pain-relieving quality. In addition, these products may reduce joint inflammation as they're absorbed into the skin. Examples include Bengay, Aspercreme, Mobisyl and Sportscreme.
- *Chili pepper seed rubs.* The seeds contain a compound called capsaicin, which causes the burning sensation. Creams made with capsaicin are most effective for arthritis pain in joints close to the skin surface, such as your fingers, knees and elbows. Examples include Capzasin and Zostrix.

Home remedies

Treatments for arthritis include:

Rest
If you're experiencing pain or inflammation in a joint, rest it for 12 to 24 hours. Do activities that don't require you to use the joint repetitively. Try taking a 10-minute break every hour.

Exercise
Exercise is probably the one therapy that will do the most good for managing arthritis. Different types of exercise can achieve different goals. For better flexibility, try gentle stretching. Brisk walking, bicycling, swimming and dancing are good examples of aerobic exercise that puts low to moderate amounts of stress on your joints.

Don't continue any exercise beyond the point that's painful without the advice of your doctor.

Heat and cold
Both heat and cold can relieve joint pain. Heat also relieves stiffness, and cold can relieve muscle spasms. Apply heat for 20 minutes several times a day using a heating pad, hot water bottle or warm bath. Cool joint pain with cold treatments, such as with ice packs. You can use cold treatments several times a day, but don't use them if you have poor circulation or numbness.

Many people with rheumatoid arthritis find relief by soaking their joints in warm water for four minutes and then in cool water for a minute. Repeat the cycle for a half-hour, ending with a warm-water soak.

Lose weight
Being overweight or obese increases the stress on weight-bearing joints, such as your knees and hips. Managing even a small amount of weight loss can relieve some pressure and reduce pain.

Relaxation
Relaxation techniques such as hypnosis, visualization, deep breathing, muscle relaxation and others may help decrease joint pain.

Tai chi and yoga
These movement therapies involve gentle stretches combined with deep breathing. Several small studies have found they may help relieve osteoarthritic pain. Avoid any movements that cause pain.

Glucosamine and chondroitin
Glucosamine and chondroitin are natural compounds found in cartilage. Supplements of both compounds are used to treat osteoarthritis, and individuals with severe symptoms seem to benefit the most. Although long-term effectiveness requires further study, glucosamine and chondroitin may help and appear to be safe, so it may not hurt to give them a try.

Asthma

Asthma occurs when the main air passages of your lungs (bronchial tubes) become inflamed and constricted, or narrowed. The muscles in the bronchial walls tighten, and the passageways produce extra mucus, reducing the flow of air.

Common signs and symptoms are wheezing, shortness of breath, chest tightness and coughing. In emergencies, you may have extreme difficulty breathing, a high pulse rate, sweating and severe coughing.

Millions of Americans — adults and children — have asthma. It isn't clear why some people get asthma and others don't, but it's probably due to a combination of environmental and genetic (inherited) factors.

Common asthma triggers

A family history of asthma, frequent childhood respiratory infections, exposure to secondhand smoke and a low birth weight may increase your risk of developing asthma. Common triggers of asthma attacks include:

- Air pollutants such as smoke or fumes
- Chemical smells
- Cockroaches
- Cold air or air conditioning
- Colds or flu (influenza)
- Dust or dust mites
- Exercise, physical activity or sports
- Foods, such as peanuts or shellfish
- Heartburn
- Medications, such as aspirin or beta blockers
- Menstrual cycle
- Mold or mildew
- Perfume or deodorant
- Pet allergy
- Stress or strong emotional reactions, such as crying
- Sulfites (preservatives in some foods and beverages)
- Tobacco smoke
- Weather, such as high humidity

Medical help

See your doctor if you think that you have asthma or if your symptoms or lung function (peak flow) readings seem to be getting worse. In case of a severe asthma attack, seek emergency medical help.

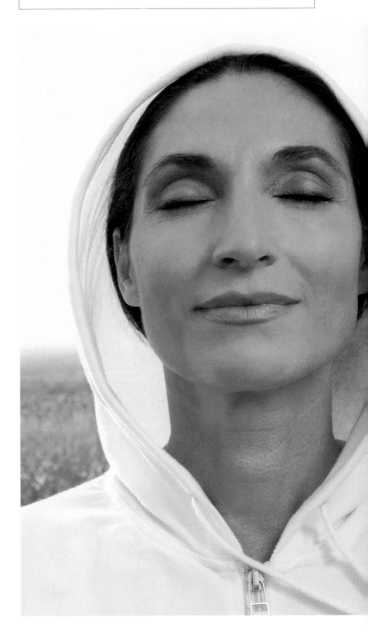

Home remedies

These tips can help control your asthma symptoms by trigger proofing your environment:

- *Avoid allergens that might be causing your symptoms.* If you're allergic to cats or dogs, consider removing them from your home and avoid contact with other people's pets. Avoid buying clothing, furniture or rugs made from animal hair.
- *Use your air conditioner.* Air conditioning helps reduce the amount of airborne pollen from trees, grasses and weeds that somehow finds its way indoors. Air conditioning also lowers indoor humidity and can reduce your exposure to dust mites. If you don't have air conditioning installed in your house, keep your windows closed during pollen season and use a fan.
- *Check your furnace.* If you have a forced-air heating system and you're allergic to dust, use a filter for dust control. Change or clean filters on heating and cooling units monthly. The best filter is a high-efficiency particulate air (HEPA) filter. Wear a mask when you remove dirty filters.
- *Clean weekly.* Avoid dust buildups in your house. Use a vacuum cleaner with a small-particle filter. Avoid projects that raise dust.
- *Don't smoke, and avoid secondhand smoke.* Avoid all types of smoke, even the type from a fireplace or burning leaves. Smoke irritates the eyes, nose and bronchial tubes.
- *Avoid activities that might contribute to your symptoms.* For example, home improvement projects might expose you to triggers that lead to an asthma attack, such as paint vapors, wood dust, mold or similar irritants.

Exercise

Years ago if you had asthma, doctors told you not to exercise. Now they believe well-planned regular workouts are beneficial, especially if you have mild to moderate symptoms. If you're fit, your heart and lungs don't have to work as hard to expel air.

However, because vigorous exercise can trigger an attack, make sure you choose suitable activities and exercise at a moderate pace. Consider talking with your doctor about an appropriate exercise schedule.

Maintain a healthy weight

Being overweight can worsen asthma symptoms, and the excess pounds put you at higher risk of other health problems.

Control heartburn and GERD

It's possible that the acid reflux causing your heartburn may also be damaging your lungs and worsening asthma symptoms. Avoid foods, beverages or activities, including overeating, that seem to cause heartburn. If your heartburn is frequent or constant, discuss treatment options with your doctor. You may need treatment for gastroesophageal reflux disease (GERD) before your asthma symptoms improve.

Athlete's foot

Athlete's foot is a fungal infection that develops between your toes and sometimes on other parts of your foot. Mold-like fungi called dermatophytes cause athlete's foot. These fungi live on the outer layer of your skin.

Dermatophytes thrive in moist, closed environments created by thick, tight shoes that squeeze the toes together, creating warm areas between them. Damp socks and shoes and warm, humid conditions also favor the organisms' growth. Plastic shoes in particular provide a welcoming environment for fungal infection.

Athlete's foot usually causes itching, stinging and burning with redness, especially between your toes. Sometimes the sole and sides of the foot are affected, appearing thickened and leathery in texture. Sections of skin may become excessively dry and cracked.

Although locker rooms and public showers are often blamed for spreading athlete's foot, the environment inside your shoes is probably more important. Athlete's foot becomes more common with age.

Medical help

See a doctor if your symptoms last longer than four weeks or they worsen. Seek medical help sooner if you notice excessive redness, swelling, drainage or fever. In addition, if you have diabetes and suspect you have athlete's foot, see your doctor.

Home remedies

To manage and prevent athlete's foot:
- *Treat your feet.* Try over-the-counter antifungal creams (Lotrimin AF, Tinactin, others) or a drying powder two to three times a day until the rash disappears.
- *Keep your feet dry.* This is particularly important for the areas between your toes. Go barefoot to let your feet air out as much as possible when you're home.
- *Wear well-ventilated shoes.* Avoid shoes made of synthetic materials, especially ones that are tightly closed.
- *Alternate shoes.* Don't wear the same shoes every day, and don't store them in plastic. Dry shoes immediately if they become wet.
- *Wear waterproof sandals or shoes.* Do this around public pools and showers and in locker rooms where infection can spread.
- *Don't borrow shoes.* Borrowing risks spreading a fungal infection.
- *Wear good socks.* Buy socks that are made of natural material, such as cotton or wool, or a synthetic fiber designed to draw moisture away from your feet. If your feet sweat a lot, change socks twice a day.

Back pain

Almost everyone has a back problem at some point in his or her lifetime. Muscle tone and strength tend to decrease with age, making your back more prone to injury.

Your spine may stiffen, the intervertebral disks wear out, and the spaces between the vertebrae narrow, allowing bone to rub on bone. These changes are common but don't have to be painful.

Back pain also may result from an injury, strain or overdoing an activity. Often, it's hard to pinpoint the cause of back pain due to the back's complex structure.

Because your lower back carries most of your weight, it tends to be the site of most back pain. However, sprains and strains can injure any part of your back.

Common causes

Causes of back pain include:
- Improper lifting
- Sudden, strenuous physical effort
- Trauma from an accident, fall or sports injury
- Lack of muscle tone
- Excess weight, especially around your middle
- Daily stress and tension
- Sleeping position, especially if you sleep on your stomach
- Poor sitting and standing postures
- Sitting in one position for a long time or with a thick wallet in your back pocket
- Carrying a heavy briefcase, shoulder bag or backpack
- Holding a forward-bending position for a long time
- Relaxation of muscles and ligaments during pregnancy

Listen up!

When your back starts hurting, it's warning you to slow down to prevent further injury.

A severe muscle spasm may last 48 to 72 hours, followed by several days or weeks of less severe pain. Most back pain disappears within a few weeks. Even after you start feeling a little better, strenuous use of the muscle during the three to six weeks after the initial injury may continue causing pain.

Regular exercise to maintain your flexibility and strength and to keep your abdominal muscles strong are your best bets to avoid back problems.

Medical help

Although uncommon, back pain can result from serious problems such as cancer, inflammatory arthritis and other diseases. Pain that worsens or remains constant for a month or more should be investigated by a doctor. Seek medical care immediately if your pain:
- Is severe, progressive or prolonged (lasting more than a month).
- Results from an injury. Don't try to move someone who has severe pain or can't move his or her arms or legs after an accident.
- Produces weakness, pain or numbness in your legs or arms.
- Is new and accompanied by an unexplained fever or weight loss.
- Is constant and worse at night.
- Is accompanied by poorly controlled blood pressure, abdominal aortic aneurysm, cancer, or sudden loss of bowel or bladder control.

Home remedies

Healing occurs most quickly if you're able to continue with your daily routine in a gentle manner and at the same time avoid any movements or actions that may have initially caused the back pain.

With proper care of a strain or sprain, you should improve within the first two weeks. Most forms of acute back pain improve in four to six weeks. Sprained ligaments or severe muscle strains may take up to 12 weeks to heal.

Apply ice

Use cold packs initially to relieve pain. Wrap an ice pack or a bag of frozen vegetables in cloth. Hold it on the sore area for 15 minutes and repeat every two to three hours. To avoid frostbite, never place ice directly on your skin.

Rest up, but move

Getting plenty of rest allows your back to heal, but avoid prolonged bed rest — lying in bed for more than a day or two may actually slow recovery. Moderate movement helps keep your muscles strong. Avoid the activity that caused the injury. Avoid lifting, pushing, pulling, repetitive bending and twisting.

Stretch

Do gentle stretching exercises. Avoid jerking, bouncing, or any movements that increase pain or require straining. Spending 10 to 15 minutes a day doing gentle exercises also can help prevent back problems (see page 22).

Get a massage

If back pain is caused by tense or overworked muscles, massage may help loosen knotted muscles and promote relaxation.

Progressive relaxation

This relaxation technique involves systematically tensing and relaxing different muscle groups in your body. Progressive relaxation boosts your ability to recognize and counteract muscle tension as soon as it starts.

Yoga

Studies indicate that yoga can help relieve back pain, with the improvement in symptoms lasting several months.

Stand, sit and lift smart

Stand up straight. Don't stand with your shoulders and back hunched. Sit up straight, with your lower back against the back of the chair. Use chairs that support your lower back. When lifting, let your legs do the work. Bend at the knees and keep your back straight.

Apply heat

After 48 hours, or once the swelling is gone, you may use heat to relax sore or knotted muscles. Use a warm bath, warm packs, heating pad or heat lamp. Be careful not to burn your skin with extreme heat. If you find that applying cold provides more relief than heat does, continue using cold, or try a combination of the two methods.

Cold versus hot

When do you apply cold and when do you apply heat to treat an injury?

	Cold	Hot
What it does	Cold reduces inflammation, constricts blood vessels to limit bruising and relieves pain by acting as a local anesthetic.	Heat improves circulation to speed healing, reduces pain by relaxing tight or sore muscles, and helps restore range of motion.
When to use it	Use cold for one to three days after an injury. Apply cold for 15 minutes at a time, every two to three hours.	Use heat once the swelling is gone. Apply heat for 20 minutes at a time, several times a day.

Daily back exercises

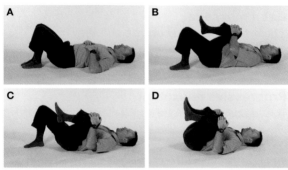

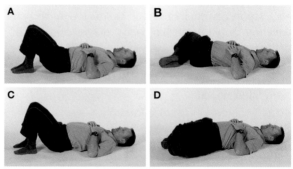

Knee-to-chest stretch

Lie on your back with your knees bent and your feet flat on the floor (A). Using both hands, pull up one knee and press it to your chest (B). Hold for 15 to 30 seconds. Return to the starting position and repeat with the opposite leg (C). Return to the starting position and repeat with both legs at the same time (D).

Lower back rotational stretch

Lie on your back with your knees bent and your feet flat on the floor (A). Keeping your shoulders firmly on the floor, roll your bent knees to one side (B). Hold for five to 10 seconds. Return to the starting position (C). Repeat on the opposite side (D).

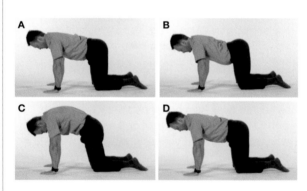

Shoulder blade squeeze

Sit on an armless chair or stool (A). Keeping your chin tucked in and your chest high, pull your shoulder blades together (B). Hold for five seconds, then relax. Repeat.

Cat stretch

Position yourself on your hands and knees (A). Slowly let your back and abdomen sag toward the floor (B). Then slowly arch your back, as if you're pulling your abdomen up toward the ceiling (C). Return to the starting position. Repeat (D).

Bad breath

There are many causes of bad breath. Your mouth itself may be a source. The breakdown of food particles and other debris by bacteria in and around your teeth can cause a foul odor.

If your mouth becomes dry, such as occurs during sleep or after smoking, dead cells can accumulate and decompose on your tongue, gums and cheeks, causing odor.

Eating foods containing oils with a strong odor, such as onions and garlic, can lead to bad breath. Foul-smelling breath may also be a symptom of illness, such as lung disease, diabetes or liver failure.

Medical help

If your breath is still bad after trying the approaches in the box at right, talk to your doctor or dentist.

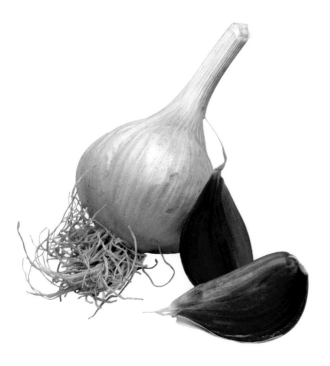

Home remedies

The following steps may help improve or prevent bad breath:

- *Brush your teeth after you eat.* Keep a toothbrush at work to brush after eating. Be sure to brush at least twice a day for two to three minutes at a time.
- *Brush your tongue.* Give your tongue a gentle brushing to remove dead cells, bacteria and food debris. Use a soft-bristled toothbrush or flexible tongue scraper. Try to clean as far back as you can because bacteria tend to collect toward the back of your mouth.
- *Floss daily.* Proper flossing removes food particles and plaque from between your teeth.
- *Clean your dentures well.* If you wear a bridge or a partial or complete denture, clean it thoroughly at least once a day or as directed by your dentist.
- *Avoid strong foods that cause bad breath.* These include onions, garlic and hot peppers. The odors from these types of foods generally linger in your mouth.
- *Drink plenty of water.* To keep your mouth moist, be sure to consume plenty of water, and not coffee, soft drinks or alcohol.
- *Grab some gum or a mint.* Chewing a piece of gum (preferably sugarless) or sucking on candy (preferably sugarless) stimulates saliva, washing away food particles and bacteria. If you have chronic dry mouth, your dentist or doctor may prescribe an artificial saliva preparation or an oral medication that stimulates the flow of saliva.
- *Chew fresh parsley.* Chewing on parsley may temporarily improve bad breath.

Bedbugs

Bedbugs have feasted on sleeping humans for thousands of years. After World War II, they were eradicated from most developed nations with the use of DDT. This pesticide has since been banned because it's so toxic to the environment.

Spurred perhaps by an increase in international travel, bedbugs are becoming a problem once again. The risk of encountering bedbugs increases if you spend time in locations with a high turnover of nighttime guests — such as hotels, hospitals or homeless shelters.

Bedbugs are small, reddish brown, oval and flat. During the day, they hide in the cracks and crevices of beds, box springs, headboards and bed frames.

What to look for

It can be difficult to distinguish bedbug bites from other kinds of insect bites. In general, bedbug bites are:
- Red, often with a darker red spot in the middle
- Itchy
- Arranged in a rough line or in a cluster
- Located on the face, neck, arms and hands

Some people have no reaction at all to bedbug bites, while others experience an allergic reaction that may include severe itching, blisters or hives.

Medical help

If you experience allergic reactions or severe skin reactions to your bedbug bites, see your doctor.

Home remedies

The redness and itching associated with bedbug bites usually goes away within a week or two. You might speed recovery by using:
- Skin cream containing hydrocortisone
- Oral antihistamine, such as diphenhydramine (Benadryl)

Treating your home

Once your symptoms are treated, you must tackle the underlying infestation. This can be difficult because bedbugs hide well and can live for months without eating. Nonchemical treatments include:
- *Vacuuming.* A thorough vacuuming of cracks and crevices can physically remove bedbugs from an area. But vacuum cleaners can't reach all hiding places.
- *Hot water.* Washing clothes and other items in water that's at least 120 F can kill bedbugs.
- *Clothes dryer.* Placing sheets, pillowcases and other bedding in a clothes dryer set at medium to high heat for 20 minutes will kill bedbugs and their eggs.
- *Enclosed vehicle.* If it's summer, bag up infested items and leave them in a car parked in the sun with the windows rolled up for a day. The target temperature is at least 120 F.
- *Freezing.* Bedbugs are vulnerable to temperatures below 32 F, but you'd need to leave the bedding and other items outdoors or in the freezer for several days.

Prevention

To prevent infestations and bites:
- *Inspect secondhand items.* Check used mattresses or upholstered furniture carefully before bringing it into your home.
- *Use hotel precautions.* Check mattress seams for bedbug excrement, and don't place your luggage on the floor.
- *Cover up.* Because bedbugs don't tend to burrow under clothing, you may be able to avoid bites by wearing long pajamas.

Bed-wetting

Bed-wetting isn't a sign of toilet training gone bad. It's often just a childhood developmental stage.

Generally, bed-wetting before age 6 or 7 should not be a cause for concern. At this age, nighttime bladder control simply may not be established.

If bed-wetting continues past age 7, treat the concern with patience and understanding. Bladder training, moisture alarms and other steps may help reduce bed-wetting.

Often, bed-wetting occurs for simple reasons, such as forgetting to go to the bathroom before bedtime. Other causes may include stress, constipation or an inability to recognize when the bladder is full.

Several underlying factors associated with the increased risk of bed-wetting include:

- **Sex.** Bed-wetting is more common in boys than in girls.
- **Family history.** If both parents wet the bed as children, their child has an increased risk of wetting the bed.
- **Attention-deficit/hyperactivity disorder (ADHD).** Bed-wetting is more common in children who have ADHD.

Medical help

Most children outgrow bed-wetting on their own, but sometimes bed-wetting may indicate an underlying condition that requires medical attention. Consult your child's doctor if:

- Your child regularly wets the bed after age 7
- Your child starts wetting the bed after a period of being dry at night
- The bed-wetting is accompanied by painful urination, unusual thirst, pink urine or snoring

Home remedies

Changes you can make at home that may reduce bed-wetting include:

- *Limit your child's fluid intake in the evening.* Around 8 ounces or so of fluid in the evening is generally enough, but be careful when you limit fluid intake for yourself or your child. Some experts feel a good approximation is for children to have 40 percent of their daily fluids between 7 a.m. and noon, another 40 percent between noon and 5 p.m. and just 20 percent after 5 p.m. However, don't limit fluids if your child participates in evening sports, either practices or games. Check with your doctor to find out what's right for your child.
- *Avoid caffeinated drinks and foods in the evening.* Caffeine may increase the need to urinate, so don't give your child caffeinated drinks, such as cola, or snacks, such as chocolate, in the evening.
- *Encourage double voiding before bed.* Double voiding is urinating at the beginning of the bedtime routine, for example, before changing into pajamas — and then again just before lights out. Remind your child that it's OK to use the toilet during the night if needed. Use small night lights so that your child can easily find the way between the bedroom and the bathroom.
- *Encourage regular urination throughout the day.* During awake hours, suggest that your child urinate once every two hours, or at least enough to avoid a feeling of urgency.
- *Treat constipation.* If constipation is a problem for your child, treating that problem may also reduce bed-wetting.
- *Experiment with foods.* Some people believe that certain foods negatively affect bladder function and that removing these foods from your child's diet may decrease bed-wetting. More study on this idea is necessary. However, if you think a food may be a problem, avoid it for awhile (only one food at a time) and see what happens.

Black eye

An injury or trauma to the face or head may cause bleeding beneath the skin around your eye.

The so-called black eye is due to discoloration from the collected blood as well as swelling of the soft tissue around the eye socket.

Most black eyes are not serious injuries, and the eye itself is usually not damaged. Generally, a black eye heals within a few days. However, it may indicate a more extensive injury, even a skull fracture — particularly if the area around both eyes is bruised or there has been head trauma.

Sometimes, there's an accompanying injury to the eyeball that's sufficient to cause bleeding within the eye. This condition, called a hyphema, can be serious, reducing vision and damaging the cornea. For this reason, it's advisable to have an eye specialist examine your eyeball if there has been enough of an injury to cause a black eye.

Medical help

Seek medical care immediately if you experience vision problems (double vision, blurring), severe pain, bleeding in the eye or from the nose, or loss of consciousness.

Home remedies

To reduce bruising and swelling around the eye:
- Using gentle pressure, apply ice or a cold pack to the area around the eye for 15 minutes several times a day. Apply cold as soon as possible after the injury. Don't apply ice directly to your skin — first wrap it in a small towel or washcloth.
- Take care not to press on the eye itself when you're applying ice or cleaning the area around the injury.
- Continue using ice or cold packs for 24 to 48 hours.
- Take acetaminophen (Tylenol, others) for pain associated with the black eye. Don't take aspirin, which may delay blood from clotting and make the bruised area even larger.

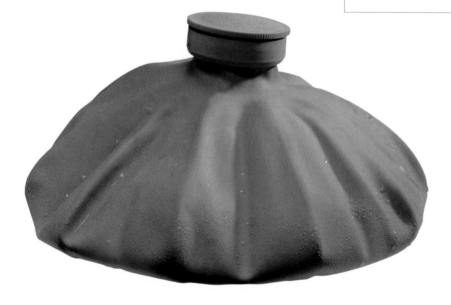

Bladder infection

Bladder infections, also known as urinary tract infections (UTIs), are usually caused by bacteria that have entered the tract from the anal region. The condition is common among women, especially in their reproductive years.

Your urinary system is composed of the kidneys, ureters, bladder and urethra. Any part of your urinary system can become infected, but most infections involve the lower urinary tract — the urethra and the bladder.

With the beginning of sexual activity, women have a marked increase in the number of infections. Sexual intercourse, pregnancy and urinary obstruction all contribute to the likelihood of such an infection.

Signs and symptoms include pain or a burning sensation during urination, an increase in the number of times you need to urinate, and a feeling of urgency every time you urinate.

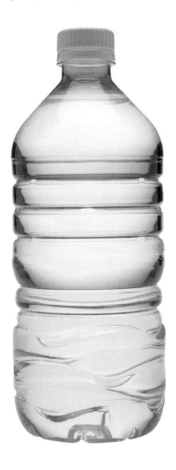

Medical help

If you have symptoms of a bladder infection, contact your doctor.

Home remedies

The following steps may ease the discomfort of a bladder infection until antibiotics prescribed by your doctor can clear the infection:

- *Drink plenty of water.* Water dilutes your urine and helps flush out bacteria. Avoid coffee, alcohol, and soft drinks containing citrus juices and caffeine until your infection has cleared. These kinds of beverages may irritate your bladder and increase the frequency or urgency of urination.
- *Use a heating pad.* Place the pad on your abdomen at low to moderate heat to minimize bladder pressure or discomfort. If you don't have a heating pad, a hot water bottle or washcloth soaked in hot water may work just as well.

Prevention

Take these steps to reduce your risk of a bladder infection:

- *Drink plenty of liquids.* Water is best to flush bacteria from your urinary tract, reducing the risk of infection.
- *Wipe from front to back.* Doing so after urinating and after a bowel movement helps prevent bacteria in the anal region from spreading to the vagina and urethra.
- *Go to the bathroom as soon as possible after intercourse.* Emptying your bladder helps flush bacteria from your urinary tract.
- *Avoid potentially irritating feminine products.* Using deodorant sprays or other feminine products, such as douches and powders, in the genital area can irritate the urethra.

Blisters

A blister is a pocket of fluid that forms under your skin, commonly caused by friction or rubbing, burning, or freezing. The blister can be painful, especially when pressure is applied to the site.

To reduce risk of infection, try keeping the pocket intact. Unbroken skin over a blister provides a natural barrier to bacteria. Don't puncture a blister unless it's very painful or it prevents you from walking or using your hands.

Cover a small blister with an adhesive bandage, and cover a large one with a porous, plastic-coated gauze pad that absorbs moisture and allows the wound to breathe.

You may protect a small intact blister with moleskin — a soft, plush fabric with adhesive backing that's sold in many drugstores and pharmacies. Cut a piece of moleskin into a doughnut shape and place the pad so that it encircles the blister, with the open center directly over the blister pocket. Then cover the blister and moleskin with gauze. The moleskin and gauze will cushion the blister and protect it from further friction and rubbing.

Medical help

Call your doctor if you see signs or symptoms of infection around a blister — pus, redness, increasing pain or warm skin. If you have diabetes or poor circulation, call your doctor before treating the blister yourself.

Home remedies

Priorities in the treatment of blisters are avoiding the source of friction or rubbing and then protecting the injury until your skin has had time to heal.

To relieve blister-related pain, drain the fluid while leaving the overlying skin intact. Here's how:

- *Prepare first.* Wash your hands and the blister site with soap and warm water. Swab the blister with iodine or rubbing alcohol. Sterilize a clean, sharp needle by wiping it with rubbing alcohol.
- *Use the needle to puncture the blister.* Aim for several spots near the blister's edge. Let the fluid drain, but leave the overlying skin in place.
- *Protect the area.* Apply an antibiotic ointment to the blister and cover with a bandage or gauze pad.
- *Follow-up care.* Cut away all the dead skin after several days, using tweezers and scissors sterilized with rubbing alcohol. Apply more ointment and a bandage.

Shoe-shopping tips

Poorly fitting shoes are a common cause of blisters on the feet. Remember the following when you shop for shoes:

- *Shop during the middle of the day.* Your feet swell throughout the day, so a late-day fitting will probably give you the best fit.
- *Remember socks.* Wear the same socks you'll wear when walking, or bring them with you to the store.
- *Measure your feet.* Shoe sizes change throughout adulthood.
- *Measure both feet and try on both shoes.* If your feet differ in size, buy the larger size.
- *Think of support.* Go for flexible, but supportive, shoes with cushioned insoles.
- *Leave toe room.* Be sure that you can comfortably wiggle your toes.
- *Avoid shoes with seams in the toe box.* These may irritate bunions or hammertoes.

Boils

A boil is a skin infection that often appears suddenly as a painful pink or red bump, generally between ½ inch to ¾ inch in diameter. The surrounding skin may be red and swollen.

Boils usually form when one or more hair follicles become infected with staph bacteria (*Staphylococcus aureus*). The bacteria, which normally inhabit your skin's surface, may enter through a cut, scratch or other break in your skin.

Within a few days, the bump fills with pus. It grows larger and more painful, sometimes reaching golf ball size before developing a yellow-white tip that finally ruptures and drains.

Boils usually clear completely in a couple of weeks, though it can take a month or more. Small boils generally heal without scarring, but a large boil may leave a scar.

Boils can occur anywhere on your skin, but appear mainly on your face, neck, armpits, buttocks or thighs — hair-bearing areas where you're most likely to sweat or experience friction.

Medical help

Contact your doctor if the infection is located on your spine, groin or face, worsens rapidly or causes severe pain, isn't gone within two weeks, or is accompanied by a fever or reddish lines that radiate out from the boil.

Home remedies

To avoid spreading infection from a boil and to minimize discomfort, follow these measures:

- *Soak the area with a warm washcloth or compress.* Do this for at least 10 minutes every few hours. Doing so may help the boil burst and drain much sooner. Use warm salt water. (Add 1 teaspoon of salt to 1 quart of boiling water and let it cool.) Prevent the drained matter from contacting other areas of skin.
- *Gently wash the boil two to three times a day with antibacterial soap.* Then apply an over-the-counter antibiotic ointment and cover with a bandage.
- *Never squeeze or lance a boil.* You might spread the infection.
- *Wash your hands thoroughly after treating a boil.* Also, launder towels, compresses and clothing that have touched the infected area.

Breast tenderness

Generalized tenderness in both breasts may be common for many women, especially during the week before a menstrual period. These changes can be a symptom of premenstrual syndrome (see page 142). Breast tenderness may also be caused by vigorous exercise or by an inflamed cyst.

If redness develops in breast tissue and a fever occurs, then infection of the breast (mastitis) is a concern. The infection usually occurs in only one breast. Mastitis most commonly affects women who are breast-feeding.

Medical help

Breast tenderness alone rarely signifies breast cancer. Still, if you have unexplained breast pain that persists for more than a couple of weeks, causes worry about breast cancer or otherwise disrupts your life, get checked by your doctor. Also see your doctor if tenderness is associated with a lump or change in breast texture.

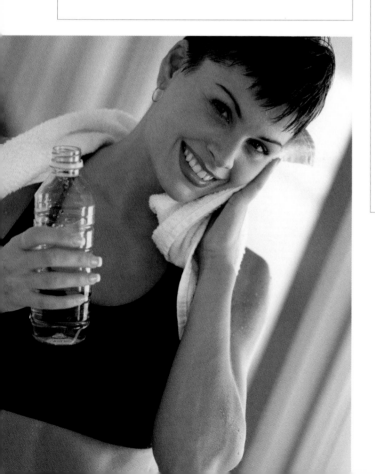

Home remedies

To reduce breast tenderness:

- *Use hot or cold compresses on your breasts.*
- *Wear a firm support bra.* Have it fitted by a professional if possible.
- *Wear a sports bra during exercise and while sleeping.* This may be especially beneficial when your breasts are more sensitive.
- *Experiment with relaxation therapy.* This can help control the high levels of anxiety associated with severe breast pain.
- *Limit or eliminate caffeine.* This is a dietary change many women swear by, although medical studies of caffeine's effect on breast pain and other premenstrual symptoms have been inconclusive.
- *Decrease the amount of fat in your diet.* Aim for less than 20 percent of total calories. This may help relieve breast pain by altering the fatty acid balance.
- *Use a pain reliever.* Nonprescription options such as acetaminophen (Tylenol, others) or ibuprofen (Advil, Motrin IB, others) may help alleviate breast pain.
- *Though not proved, vitamins and dietary supplements may lessen breast pain.* Evening primrose oil appears to change the balance of fatty acids in your cells, which may reduce breast pain. Studies of vitamin E show a possible beneficial effect on breast pain, but the medical literature to date remains inconclusive.
- *See other tips in the section on premenstrual syndrome (page 143).*

Bronchitis

Bronchitis is an inflammation of the lining of your bronchial tubes, which carry air to and from your lungs. It's usually caused by a viral infection, producing a deep cough that, in turn, brings up yellowish-gray matter from your lungs.

A common condition, acute bronchitis often develops from a cold or other respiratory infection. Chronic bronchitis, a more serious condition, is a constant irritation or inflammation of the bronchi, often due to smoking.

Signs and symptoms of bronchitis may include:
- Cough
- Production of mucus, either clear or white, or yellowish gray or green in color
- Shortness of breath, made worse by mild exertion
- Wheezing
- Fatigue
- Slight fever and chills
- Chest discomfort

Medical help

Short-lived (acute) bronchitis usually disappears in a matter of days. Contact a doctor if you experience shortness of breath or a fever of 101 F or higher for more than three days. If your cough lasts for more than 10 days with no end in sight, seek medical attention.

Home remedies

Besides the basic guidelines of getting plenty of rest and drinking plenty of fluids, the following suggestions can help make you more comfortable, speed recovery, prevent complications and help control symptoms:

- *Avoid exposure to irritants, such as tobacco smoke.* Don't smoke. Wear a mask when the air is polluted or if you're exposed to irritants, such as paint or household cleaners with strong fumes.
- *Use a humidifier in your room.* Warm, moist air helps relieve coughs and loosens mucus in your airways. But be sure to clean the humidifier according to the manufacturer's recommendations to avoid the growth of bacteria and fungi in the water container.
- *Use over-the-counter medications.* To relieve pain and lower a high fever, acetaminophen (Tylenol, others) and ibuprofen (Advil, Motrin IB, others) may help.
- *Consider a face mask outside.* If cold air aggravates your cough and causes shortness of breath, put on a cold-air face mask before you go outside.
- *Try pursed-lip breathing.* If you have chronic bronchitis, you may breathe too fast. Pursed-lip breathing helps slow your breathing, and may make you feel better. Take a deep breath, then slowly breathe out through your mouth while pursing your lips (hold them as if you're going to kiss someone.) Repeat. This technique increases the air pressure in your airways.

Bruises

A bruise forms when a blow or impact breaks blood vessels near your skin's surface, allowing a small amount of blood to leak into the tissues under your skin. The trapped blood appears as a black-and-blue mark.

Symptoms may include pain and swelling. Eventually your body resorbs the blood, and the mark disappears. The color of the bruise can change to light blue or greenish yellow before returning to normal skin color.

Bruising more common with age

Some people — especially women — are more prone to bruising than are others. As you get older, several factors may contribute to increased bruising, including:

- **Aging capillaries.** Over time, the tissues supporting these vessels weaken, and capillary walls become more fragile and prone to rupture.
- **Thinning skin.** With age, your skin becomes thinner and loses some of the protective fatty layer that helps cushion your blood vessels against injury. Excessive exposure to the sun accelerates the aging process in the skin.

Medical help

These signs and symptoms may indicate a more serious problem. See your doctor if:

- You have unusually large or painful bruises — particularly if your bruises seem to develop for no known reasons
- You bruise easily and you're experiencing abnormal bleeding elsewhere, such as from your nose or gums, or you notice blood in your eyes, stool or urine
- You have no history of bruising but suddenly experience bruises

Home remedies

You can enhance healing with these techniques:

- *Elevate the injured area, if possible.* This may help reduce the amount of blood that pools in the area.
- *Apply cold.* Apply ice, cold pack or cold compress for 20 minutes at a time, several times daily for a day or two after the injury.
- *Rest the bruised area, if possible.*
- *Try pain relievers.* Consider acetaminophen (Tylenol, others) for pain relief, or ibuprofen (Advil, Motrin IB, others) to also reduce swelling.

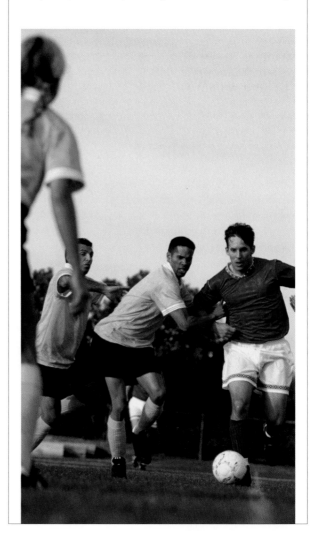

Burns

Burns are traumatic injuries, often to the outer layers of your skin, that can result from a variety of sources: fire, the sun, chemicals, hot liquids, steam electricity and other means. A burn can be a minor medical problem or a life-threatening emergency.

Treatment depends on the size and severity of the burn. Distinguishing a minor burn from a more serious burn involves understanding how much damage has occurred to the skin and underlying tissues.

The following three categories and accompanying illustrations on this page can help determine how you should respond to a burn.

First-degree burn

The least serious burns are those in which only the outer layer of skin (epidermis) is burned. The skin is usually reddened, and there may be swelling and pain, but the outer layer of skin hasn't been burned through.

Unless such a burn involves substantial portions of the hands, feet, face, groin, buttocks or a major joint, it may be treated as a minor burn with the self-care remedies listed on page 34.

Chemical burns may require additional follow-up. If the burn was caused by exposure to the sun, see "Sunburn," page 165.

Second-degree burn

When the first layer of skin has been burned through and the second layer of skin (dermis) also is burned, the injury is called a second-degree burn. Blisters form, and the skin takes on an intensely reddened, splotchy appearance. Second-degree burns usually produce swelling and moderate to severe pain.

If a second-degree burn is limited to an area no larger than 3 inches wide, follow the home remedies listed on the next page. If the burned area of the skin is larger, or if the burn is on the hands, feet, face, groin, buttocks, or over a major joint or encircles your limb, seek urgent care immediately.

Third-degree

The most serious burns involve all layers of the skin. Fat, nerves, muscles and even bones may be affected. Usually some areas are charred black or appear a dry white. There may be severe pain, or if nerve damage is substantial, no pain at all.

It's important to take quick action in all cases of third-degree burns. For more information on the treatment of severe burns while waiting for help to arrive, see page 188.

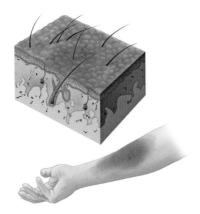

First-degree burn

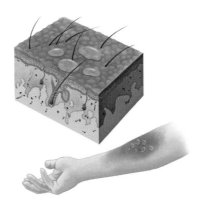

Second-degree burn

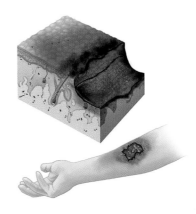

Third-degree burn

Home remedies

For minor burns, including second-degree burns limited to an area no larger than 3 inches wide, take the following actions:

Cool the burn
Hold the burned area under cold running water until the pain subsides. If this step is impractical, immerse the burn in cold water or apply cold compresses. Cooling the burn reduces pain and swelling.

Consider a lotion
Once a burn is completely cooled, applying a lotion, such as one containing aloe vera, or a moisturizer prevents drying and increases your comfort. For sunburn, try 1 percent hydrocortisone cream.

Bandage a burn
Cover the burn with a sterile gauze bandage (not fluffy cotton). Wrap it loosely to avoid putting pressure on burned skin. Bandaging keeps air off the area, reduces pain and protects blistered skin.

Take an over-the-counter pain reliever
These include aspirin, ibuprofen (Advil, Motrin IB, others), naproxen sodium (Aleve) or acetaminophen (Tylenol, others). Don't give aspirin to children younger than age 12.

Don't use ice
Applying ice on a burn can cause frostbite and do more damage.

Don't break blisters
Fluid-filled blisters protect against infection. If blisters break, clean the area daily by rinsing with water (mild soap is optional). Apply an antibiotic ointment. But if a rash appears, stop using the ointment.

Watch for signs of infection
Minor burns will usually heal in about one to two weeks without further treatment, but watch for indications of infection.

Medical help

Seek emergency medical help if the burn appears severe or covers a large area. For minor burns, see a doctor if the burn does not improve or new symptoms develop, such as a fever or lightheadedness.

Bursitis

Bursitis is a painful condition affecting small fluid-filled pads (bursae) that lubricate and cushion pressure points for your bones, tendons and muscles near your joints. Bursitis occurs when a bursa becomes inflamed.

The most common locations for bursitis are in the shoulders, elbows or hips. But you can also have bursitis at your knee, heel and base of your big toe.

Bursitis often occurs in joints that perform frequent repetitive motion. It's commonly caused by overuse, trauma, repeated bumping or prolonged pressure such as kneeling for an extended period. It may even result from an infection, arthritis or gout.

If you have bursitis, the affected joint may:
- Feel achy or stiff
- Hurt more when you move it or press on it
- Look swollen and red

Medical help

Consult your doctor if you have:
- Disabling joint pain, or pain that lasts more than two weeks
- Excessive swelling, redness, bruising or a rash in the affected area
- Sharp or shooting pain, especially when you exercise or exert yourself
- A fever that accompanies other signs and symptoms

Home remedies

To treat symptoms of bursitis:
- Use over-the-counter pain medications.
- Keep pressure off the joint. Use an elastic bandage, sling or soft foam pad to protect it until the swelling goes down.
- Ease the joint back into activity slowly.

Prevention

While not all types of bursitis can be prevented, you can reduce your risk and reduce the severity of flare-ups by changing the way you perform certain tasks. Examples include:
- *Strengthen your muscles to help protect the joint.* But don't start exercising a joint that has bursitis until the pain and inflammation are gone.
- *Warm up and stretch after.* Slowly warm up before exercise. Gently stretch after.
- *Take frequent breaks from repetitive tasks.* Alternate repetitive tasks with rest or other activities. Follow ergonomic principles for desk work and lifting.
- *Cushion the joint before applying pressure.* Use knee pads or elbow pads. For bursitis in a hip, cushion a hard mattress with a foam pad or soft mattress cover.
- *Avoid elbow pressure.* Stop leaning on your elbows. If you push up from your elbows to get out of bed, consider tying a rope to the end of your bed so that you can pull yourself up that way.
- *Lift properly.* Bend your knees when you lift. Failing to do so puts extra stress on the bursae in your hips.
- *Avoid heavy loads.* Carrying heavy loads puts stress on the bursae in your shoulders. Use a dolly instead.

Canker sores

A canker sore is an ulcer on the soft tissue inside your mouth — the tongue, soft palate, inner lips or inner cheeks. Typically, you notice a burning sensation and round whitish spot surrounded by a red edge or halo.

Despite a great deal of research on the condition, the cause of canker sores remains a mystery. Current thinking suggests that stress or tissue injury may cause the eruption of most common canker sores.

Some researchers believe certain nutritional deficiencies or food sensitivities may complicate the problem. In addition, some gastrointestinal and immune deficiency disorders have been linked to canker sores, as well as agents such as sodium lauryl sulfate — an ingredient in some brands of toothpaste.

Types

There are two types of canker sore: simple and complex. Simple canker sores may appear three or four times a year and last four to seven days. The first occurrence is usually between the ages of 10 and 40, but also can happen in younger children. As a person reaches adulthood, the sores occur less frequently. Women seem to get them more often than do men, and they seem to run in families.

Complex canker sores are less common but much more of a problem. As old sores heal, new ones appear.

Medical help

In severe cases, your dentist or doctor may recommend a prescription mouthwash, salve or solution. Contact your doctor if you have:

- Significant difficulty eating or drinking due to canker sores
- High fever with canker sores
- Spreading sores or signs of spreading infection
- Pain that's not controlled with the measures listed above
- Sores that don't heal completely within a week See your dentist if you have sharp tooth surfaces or dental appliances that are causing sores.

Home remedies

There's no cure for either simple or complex canker sores, and effective treatments are limited. To relieve pain and speed healing:

- *Rinse your mouth.* Use salt water; baking soda (dissolve 1 teaspoon of soda in 1/2 cup warm water); hydrogen peroxide diluted by half with water; or a mixture of 1 part diphenhydramine (Benadryl) to either 1 part bismuth subsalicylate (Kaopectate, Pepto-Bismol, others) or 1 part simethicone (Maalox). Be sure to spit out the mixtures after rinsing.
- *Cover lesions.* Use a paste made of baking soda and water.
- *Try over-the-counter products.* Look for ones that contain a numbing agent, such as Anbesol and Orajel.
- *Avoid abrasive, acidic or spicy foods.* They can cause further irritation and pain.
- *Apply ice to your canker sores.* Or allow ice chips to slowly dissolve over the sores.
- *Brush your teeth gently.* Use a soft brush and toothpaste without foaming agents, such as TheraBreath.
- *Try milk of magnesia.* Dab a small amount of milk of magnesia on your canker sore a few times a day. This can ease the pain and may help the sore heal more quickly.

Carpal tunnel syndrome

The carpal tunnel is a narrow passageway through your bony wrist that protects the primary nerves and tendons to your hand. When tissues in the passage become swollen or inflamed, they put pressure on a nerve that affects the sensation of your thumb and index, middle and ring fingers and the movement of your thumb. Too much pressure may cause carpal tunnel syndrome. If left untreated, permanent nerve and muscle damage can occur.

Risk factors for carpal tunnel syndrome include various occupations, activities and hobbies that involve awkward wrist positions, pressure on the palm of the hand, and repetitive lifting or grasping actions. Pregnancy, obesity and conditions such as diabetes, thyroid disease and arthritis also are risk factors.

Signs and symptoms of the condition include:

- Tingling or numbness in your thumb and index and middle fingers (but not your little finger). This sensation may occur at night, waking you up. It may also occur while you're driving or holding a phone or newspaper.
- Pain radiating or extending from your wrist up your arm to your shoulder or down into your palm or fingers, especially after forceful or repetitive use.
- Sense of weakness in your hands and a tendency to drop objects.

Medical help

If the symptoms continue for more than a couple of weeks, see your doctor. Splints, therapy, injection or prescription medications may be recommended. Occasionally, surgery is necessary.

Home remedies

To relieve carpal tunnel symptoms:

- *Take frequent breaks.* Every hour take a 5-minute break and gently stretch your wrists and hands.
- *Vary your activities.* Alternate tasks involving your hands when possible.
- *Watch your form.* Avoid bending your wrist all the way up or down.
- *Relax your grip.* Avoid using a hard grip when driving your car, bicycling or writing. Oversized grips on pens, pencils and tools may allow a softer grasp.
- *Keep your hands warm.* You're more likely to develop hand pain and stiffness if you work in a cold environment. If you can't control the temperature at work, put on fingerless gloves that keep your hands and wrists warm.
- *Use a wrist splint at night.* A wrist splint may help ease pain or numbness in your wrists and hands. The splint should be snug but not tight.
- *Use nonprescription pain relievers.* Nonsteroidal anti-inflammatory drugs (NSAIDs), such as ibuprofen (Advil, Motrin IB, others), can help relieve both pain and swelling.
- *Try yoga and other relaxation techniques.* Yoga postures designed for strengthening, stretching and balancing joints in the upper body, as well as the upper body itself, may help reduce pain and improve the grip strength of people with carpal tunnel syndrome.

Chronic pain

Physical pain is a part of life. Maybe you've slammed your finger in a door, burned your hand while touching a hot skillet on the stove or twisted your ankle while playing basketball. The result is a sensation of sharp or aching pain.

Chronic pain is persistent pain lasting long after the normal healing process, or when there doesn't seem to be any injury or bodily damage that could cause the ongoing sensation. Generally, chronic pain is considered to be pain that lasts more than three to six months.

Chronic pain can be overwhelming. But you can learn how to manage the pain so that it doesn't interfere with your life. Your outlook and positive attitude also are important.

Pain and your emotions

Pain isn't only a physical experience but also an emotional one.

People perceive pain differently and react to it in different ways. When you experience pain over a long period of time, you may find yourself overwhelmed by intense, often negative, emotions, including panic, fear, grief, anxiety and anger. Chronic pain can cause frustration and irritability. These emotions can affect you physically, sapping your energy and intensifying the symptoms.

Finding healthy ways to cope with pain can have both physical and emotional benefits.

Medical help

If your pain changes in character — for example, it grows from mild to severe — or if you develop new symptoms, such as a tingling or numb sensation, it might be a good idea to see your doctor and have your condition re-evaluated.

Pain relievers: Matching the pill to the pain

For pain relief, the difference among nonprescription pain relievers is generally more subtle than significant. All over-the-counter pain relievers relieve mild to moderate pain associated with common conditions such as headache, muscle aches and arthritis. They also reduce a fever. The difference among the various products is that some relieve inflammation while others don't:

- *NSAIDs.* These products, which include ibuprofen (Advil, Motrin IB, others) and naproxen sodium (Aleve), reduce inflammation. NSAID stands for nonsteroidal anti-inflammatory drugs. They're most helpful for pain associated with arthritis and tendinitis.
- *Acetaminophen.* The most common brand of acetaminophen is Tylenol. Acetaminophen doesn't relieve inflammation but does relieve pain.

With all nonprescription pain relievers, you need to be careful about how many you take. They all have side effects that can be serious if the medications are taken in excessive amounts.

Home remedies

There are many methods for relieving chronic pain. Experiment with different therapies to find which ones work best for you.

Exercise

Physical activity can stimulate the release of endorphins, your body's own natural painkillers. Endorphins are morphine-like pain relievers that send "stop pain" messages to your sensitive nerve cells.

The duration of exercise seems to be more important than the intensity. Low-intensity aerobic exercise — for example, brisk walking — for 30 to 45 minutes on five or six days a week may have a positive effect. (Be sure to build up slowly.) You can even benefit from only three days of exercise a week.

If you want to start an exercise program that's more vigorous than walking, have a medical evaluation, especially if:

- You're older than age 40
- You've been sedentary
- You have risk factors for coronary artery disease
- You have chronic health problems

Hot and cold

Heat and ice are used most often to treat acute pain following an injury but may also help relieve some forms of chronic pain. For more on the use of hot and cold for injury, see page 21.

Weight loss

It's easier to manage pain when you're not overweight. Excess weight saps your energy, increases stress on your muscles and joints, and decreases flexibility. You don't have to become thin, but losing just a few pounds may help reduce your pain level.

Sleep

You're better equipped to deal with pain if you've had a good night's sleep. Sleep gives you energy and helps you fight off fatigue and stress, which can worsen pain. For tips on better sleep, see pages 115-116.

Topical medications

Several medications are available without a prescription that may help relieve pain for a short time.

Capsaicin (Capzasin-P, Zostrix) is the active ingredient in nonprescription creams made from the seeds of hot chili peppers. Rub the product on your skin three to five times a day. Some people find capsaicin helpful for arthritic pain in joints close to the skin's surface, such as fingers and elbows. It may also help relieve pain after shingles. However, the cream can temporarily irritate the skin and produce a burning sensation, which may be painful.

Counterirritants, such as Bengay and Icy Hot, include ingredients such as menthol and oil of wintergreen that stimulate nerve endings to produce feelings of cold or warmth. These responses, which may be mildly painful, can counter, or block, more intense pain sensations.

Benzocaine and lidocaine are local anesthetics that deaden your nerve endings — relieving pain and itching — where the cream or gel is applied to your skin. They're both available in prescription and nonprescription options.

Stress reduction

When you're dealing with pain, you're less able to cope with the stress of everyday living. Stress may also cause you to do things that end up intensifying pain, such as tensing your muscles. In short, pain causes stress and stress tends to make pain worse.

To better manage stress, you can learn and practice various relaxation techniques, such as:

- *Relaxed breathing.* Get in a relaxed position and close your eyes. Inhale slowly to the count of six. Hold the air in your lungs as you slowly count to four. Release the air slowly through your mouth as you count to six. Repeat three to five times.
- *Meditation.* This technique appears to reduce pain and stress by helping you relax and respond to the flow of emotions and thoughts you face in challenging situations.

Massage

A growing body of literature is beginning to validate the many benefits of massage, including helping with pain relief. Studies suggest that it can decrease headache and fibromyalgia pain and, possibly, back pain.

(Continued on next page.)

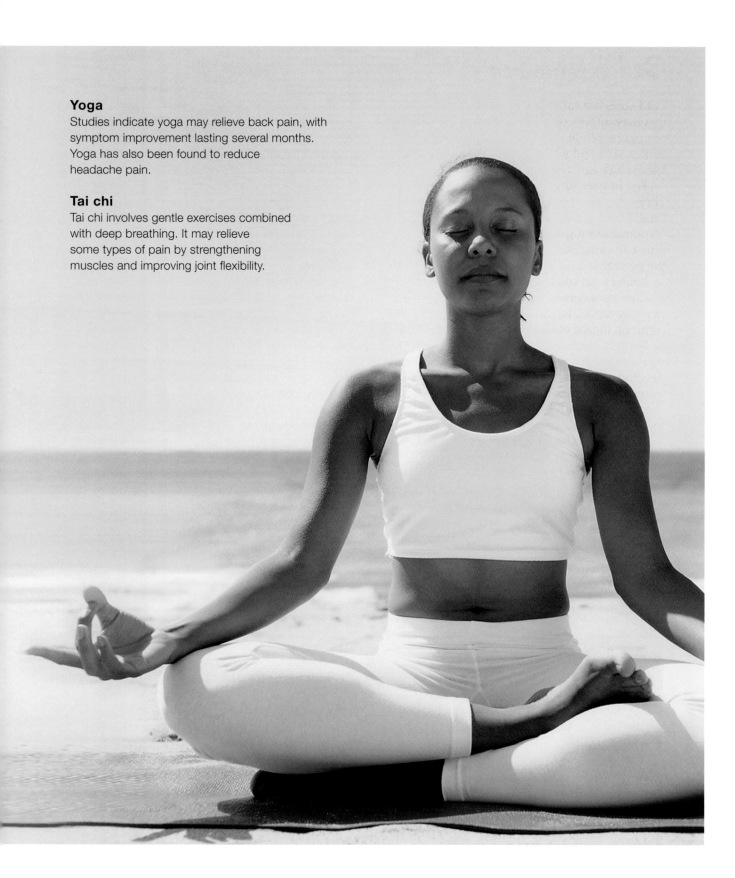

Yoga

Studies indicate yoga may relieve back pain, with symptom improvement lasting several months. Yoga has also been found to reduce headache pain.

Tai chi

Tai chi involves gentle exercises combined with deep breathing. It may relieve some types of pain by strengthening muscles and improving joint flexibility.

Cold sores

Cold sores are small, painful, fluid-filled blisters that may appear on your mouth, lips, nose, cheeks or fingers. While cold sores occur most often in adolescents and young adults, they can occur at almost any age. Outbreaks decrease after age 35.

The herpes simplex virus causes cold sores. There are two types of this virus: Type 1 usually causes cold sores, while type 2 is most often responsible for genital herpes. However, either type can cause sores in the facial area or on the genitals.

You can get cold sores from contact with another person who has an active condition. Eating utensils, razors, towels or direct skin contact are common means of spreading this infection.

Symptoms may not start for up to 20 days after you were first exposed to the virus. The blisters develop on a raised, red, painful area of skin. Pain or tingling often precedes blister formation by one to two days. Cold sores typically clear up in seven to 10 days.

After the initial infection, the virus periodically re-emerges at or near the original site. Fever, menstruation and exposure to the sun may trigger the recurrence.

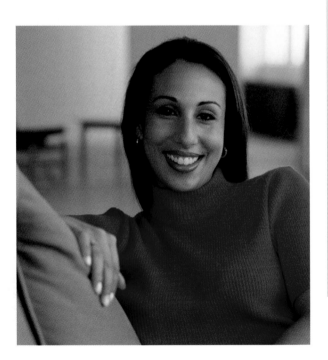

Medical help

If you have frequent bouts of cold sores, an antiviral medication may help. These medications inhibit the growth of the herpes virus. Talk to your doctor about a prescription.

Caution: If you have a cold sore, take special care to avoid contact with infants or anyone who has eczema (see page 70). A person with eczema is more susceptible to infection. Also, avoid people who are taking medications for cancer and organ transplantation because they have decreased immunity. Herpes simplex viral infections can lead to potentially serious eye complications.

Home remedies

Cold sores generally clear up without treatment. These steps may provide relief:

- *Rest and try pain relievers.* Take nonprescription pain relievers if you have a fever or the cold sore is painful. Nonprescription pain creams also may provide comfort, but they won't speed healing. Note: Children and teenagers recovering from flu-like symptoms should never take aspirin. This is because aspirin has been linked to Reye's syndrome, a rare but potentially life-threatening condition, in such children.
- *Don't squeeze, pinch or pick at any blister.*
- *Apply compresses.* Try applying ice or warm compresses to the blisters to ease pain.
- *Wash before contact.* Wash your hands carefully before touching another person. Avoid kissing and skin contact with people while blisters are present.
- *Use sunblock.* Apply on your lips and face before prolonged exposure to the sun — during winter and summer — to prevent cold sores.

Colic

Generations of families have had to deal with colic. This frustrating and largely unexplainable condition affects babies who otherwise seem healthy. Colic usually peaks at six weeks of age and disappears sometime in the baby's third to fifth month.

Although the term *colic* is used widely for any fussy baby, true colic is determined by the following factors:

- **Predictable crying episodes.** A colicky baby cries about the same time each day, usually in the late afternoon or evening. Colic episodes may last from a few minutes to three or more hours on any given day.
- **Posture changes.** Many colicky babies pull their legs to their chests, clench their fists or thrash around during episodes as if they are in pain.
- **Intense or inconsolable crying.** Colicky crying is intense and often high-pitched. The babies can be extremely difficult — if not impossible — to comfort.

It's still unclear why some babies have colic and other babies don't. There is no evidence to suggest that allergies, gas, hormones, mother's mood or particular handling of the baby causes colic. Know that baby's colic isn't anyone's fault. It's also important to take good care of yourself when you have a colicky baby, so you are able to manage your own stress level as well as possible.

Medical help

There are no medications to relieve colic. In general, consult with your doctor before giving your baby any medication. If you're worried that your baby is sick or if you or others caring for the baby are becoming frustrated or angry because of the crying, call your doctor or bring the baby to the doctor's office or emergency room.

Home remedies

If your doctor determines that your baby has colic, these measures may help you and your child find some relief:

- *Feed your baby.* If you think your baby may be hungry, try feeding. Sometimes more frequent — but smaller — feedings are helpful. Try to hold your baby as upright as possible, and burp your baby often. If you're breast-feeding, it may help to empty one breast completely before switching sides. This will give your baby more hindmilk, which is richer and potentially more satisfying than foremilk, which is present at the beginning of a feeding.
- *Offer a pacifier.* For many babies, sucking is a soothing activity. Even if you're breast-feeding, it's OK to offer a pacifier.
- *Hold your baby.* Cuddling helps some babies. Others quiet when they're held closely and swaddled in a lightweight blanket. Don't worry about spoiling your baby by holding him or her too much.
- *Keep your baby in motion.* Gently rock your baby in your arms or in an infant swing. Lay your baby tummy down on your knees and then sway your knees slowly. Take a walk with your baby, or buckle your baby in the car seat for a drive.
- *Turn up the background noise.* Some babies cry less when they hear steady background noise. When holding or rocking your baby, try making a continuous "shssss" sound. Turn on a kitchen or bathroom exhaust fan, or play soothing music or nature sounds, such as ocean waves or gentle rain. Sometimes the tick of a clock or metronome does the trick.
- *Use gentle heat or touch.* Give your baby a warm bath. Softly massage your baby, especially around the tummy.
- *Consider dietary changes.* If you breast-feed, see if eliminating certain foods from your own diet — such as dairy products, citrus fruits, spicy foods or drinks containing caffeine — has an effect on your baby's crying.

Common cold

The common cold is a viral infection of your upper respiratory tract — your nose and throat. A common cold is usually harmless, although it may not feel that way. If it's not a runny nose, sore throat and cough, it's watery eyes, sneezing and congestion — or maybe all of the above.

Most adults likely experience a cold two to four times a year. Children, especially preschoolers, may get a cold as many as six to 10 times annually.

Don't waste your money

Despite their claims, over-the-counter cold preparations won't cure a common cold or make it go away any sooner. Here's what's known about common cold remedies:

- **Pain relievers.** Products such as acetaminophen (Tylenol, others) and ibuprofen (Advil, Motrin IB, others) may relieve a fever, sore throat and headache. Overuse of these products can cause side effects. Be careful when giving acetaminophen to children because the dosing guidelines can be confusing. For instance, the infant-drop formulation is much more concentrated than is the syrup commonly used in older children. Use caution when giving aspirin to children or teenagers. Though aspirin is approved for use in children older than age 3, children and teenagers recovering from chickenpox or flu-like symptoms should never take aspirin. This is because aspirin has been linked to Reye's syndrome, a rare but potentially life-threatening condition, in such children.
- **Decongestant nasal sprays.** Adults shouldn't use decongestant drops or sprays for more than three days because prolonged use can cause chronic inflammation of the mucous membranes. And children shouldn't use decongestant drops or sprays at all. There's little evidence that they work in young children, and may cause side effects.
- **Cough syrups.** The American College of Chest Physicians strongly discourages the use of cough syrups because they don't effectively treat the underlying cause of cough due to colds. Some syrups contain ingredients that may alleviate coughing, but the amounts are too small to do much good and may actually be harmful for children. The college recommends against using over-the-counter cough syrups or cold medicines for anyone younger than age 14. The Food and Drug Administration strongly recommends against giving nonprescription cough and cold medicines to children younger than age 2.

Is it a cold or the flu?

Cold	Flu (influenza)
Runny nose, sneezing, nasal congestion	Runny nose
Sore throat (usually scratchy)	Sore throat and headache
Cough	Cough
No fever or low fever	Fever, usually over 101 F, chills
Mild fatigue	Moderate to severe fatigue and weakness
	Achy muscles and joints

Medical help

Most people recover from a common cold in about a week or two. If symptoms don't improve, see your doctor.

Home remedies

You may not cure the common cold, but you can make yourself more comfortable with these tips:

Drink lots of fluids

Water, juice and tea are all good choices. They help replace fluids lost during mucus production or a fever. Avoid alcohol and caffeine, which can cause dehydration, and cigarette smoke, which can aggravate your symptoms.

Try chicken soup

Generations of parents have spooned chicken soup into their sick children, and scientists have found that it does seem to help relieve symptoms in two ways.

First, it has anti-inflammatory properties that help reduce mucus production in your respiratory tract.

Second, it temporarily speeds up the movement of mucus through the nose, helping relieve congestion and limiting the time that viruses are in contact with the nasal lining.

Get some rest

If possible, stay home from work if you have a fever or bad cough, or are drowsy from medications. Rest is important to speeding recovery.

Adjust your room's humidity

If the air is dry, a cool-mist humidifier or vaporizer can moisten the air and help ease sinus congestion and coughing. Be sure to keep the humidifier clean, and regularly change the filter to prevent the growth of bacteria and molds.

Soothe your throat

Gargling with warm salt water several times a day or drinking warm lemon water mixed with honey may help soothe your sore throat and relieve the coughing spells.

Use saline nasal drops

Saline drops are effective, safe and nonirritating — even for children — for the relief of nasal congestion. The drops can be purchased over-the-counter in most drugstores. To use in babies, put several drops into a nostril, then immediately bulb suction that nostril.

Try andrographis

There is some evidence this Indian herb can reduce the severity and duration of upper respiratory infections. Andrographis may also reduce your risk of getting a cold. The herb seems safe when used short term.

Try echinacea

While no studies have shown that this herb can prevent a cold, there is some evidence that it can modestly relieve cold symptoms or shorten the duration of a cold. Echinacea seems most effective when taken soon after cold symptoms appear.

Get your vitamin C

Despite popular belief, there's no evidence that taking large doses of vitamin C reduces your risk of a cold. However, there's evidence that high doses of vitamin C — up to 6 grams a day — may have a small effect in reducing the duration of cold symptoms.

Consider zinc

There's some evidence that zinc lozenges taken at the beginning of a cold may help reduce symptoms. The claim that zinc nasal sprays are helpful is controversial. In general, the use of these sprays is discouraged because many people have experienced permanent loss of smell following use.

Constipation

You have constipation when you have infrequent bowel movements (generally, fewer than three stools a week), you pass hard stools, or you have to strain during bowel movements. You may feel a bloated sensation and crampy discomfort. This common problem is often improperly treated.

Constipation is a symptom, not a disease. It's the perception of difficult passage of stool. Contributing factors to constipation include: not drinking enough fluids, a diet low in fiber, irregular bowel habits, older age, lack of activity, pregnancy and illness. Some types of medication also may cause constipation.

Constipation can be extremely bothersome but is usually not serious. If it persists, however, constipation can lead to complications such as hemorrhoids and cracks in the anus (fissures).

Constipation in kids

Young children sometimes experience constipation because they neglect to take the time to use the bathroom. Toddlers may become constipated out of anxiety during toilet training. Stress also plays a role in bowel changes. However, as few as one bowel movement a week may be normal for your child.

Medical help

Contact your doctor if your constipation is severe or lasts longer than three weeks. In rare cases, constipation may signal more-serious medical conditions such as cancer and hormonal disturbances. Chronic use of certain laxatives add risk if you have heart or kidney failure.

Home remedies

To lessen your chance of constipation:

- *Eat on a regular schedule (including breakfast).* In addition, eat plenty of high-fiber foods, including fresh fruits, vegetables, whole-grain cereals and breads, flaxseed, and prunes.
- *Stay hydrated.* Drink plenty of water or other liquids to soften stool.
- *Increase physical activity.* Exercise stimulates bowel activity.
- *Don't ignore the urge to have a bowel movement.* Waiting to go can make stool more difficult to pass.
- *Know your laxatives.* The effectiveness of each type of laxative will vary from person to person. In general, bulk-forming laxatives, or fiber supplements, such as Citrucel and Metamucil, are the gentlest on your body and the safest to use long term. Stimulant laxatives such as Ex-lax and Senokot are the harshest and not for long-term use. However, use of any laxative, unless prescribed, can be habit-forming.
- *Don't rely on laxatives.* Overuse of certain laxatives can be harmful and make constipation worse. Overuse can cause your body to flush out vitamins and other nutrients before they're properly absorbed, and interfere with other medications you're taking. Excessive use can also cause a condition in which your bowels don't function properly and rely on laxatives for stimulation (lazy bowel syndrome).

Remedies for kids

Have your child drink plenty of fluids to soften stools. Warm baths also may help relax your child and encourage bowel movements. A diet rich in high-fiber foods, such as beans, whole grains, fruits and vegetables, will help your child's body form soft, bulky stools. Limit foods that have little or no fiber, such as cheese, meat and processed foods.

Corns and calluses

Corns and calluses are thick, hardened layers of skin that develop as your skin tries to protect itself against friction and pressure. They typically appear on your hands and feet.

Corns are small and often cone shaped with a hard center surrounded by inflamed skin. They tend to develop on parts of your feet that don't bear weight, such as the tops or sides of your toes. Corns can be painful when pressure is applied to them.

Calluses usually develop on the soles of your feet, on the palms of your hands or on your knees. Calluses are rarely painful and vary in size and shape. They're often larger than corns.

Although corns and calluses can be unsightly, treatment may be necessary only if they cause discomfort. For most people, eliminating the source of friction or pressure will help corns and calluses disappear. Both can look similar to a wart, so ask your doctor if you're not sure.

Medical help

If a corn or callus becomes very painful or inflamed, contact your doctor.

Home remedies

To relieve symptoms and prevent corns and calluses from forming:

- *Wear properly fitted shoes with adequate toe room.* Have a shoe store stretch your shoes at any point that rubs or pinches your feet. Place pads under your heels if your shoes rub. Try using a shoe insert to cushion or soften the corn while wearing shoes.
- *Wear padded gloves when using hand tools.* Or try padding your tool handles with cloth tape or covers.
- *Soak your hands or feet.* Soaking your hands or feet in warm, soapy water softens corns and calluses. This makes it easier to remove the thickened skin.
- *Use a pumice stone.* During or after bathing, rub your corn or callus with a pumice stone, metal nail file or washcloth to gradually thin some of the thickened skin. This advice isn't recommended if you have diabetes or poor circulation.
- *Try corn dissolvers containing salicylic acid.* These over-the-counter products are available as plaster-pad disks or solutions.
- *Trim corns and calluses carefully.* Don't cut or shave them with a sharp edge.
- *Use a moisturizer.* Apply moisturizing cream daily to your hands and feet to keep them soft.

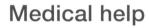

Cough

A cough is a reflex — just like breathing. It's actually a way of protecting your lungs against irritants, such as dust or smoke. When there's a buildup of fine particles or mucus in your breathing passages (bronchi), you cough to clear the passages, allowing easier breathing.

A small amount of coughing is normal and even healthy as a way to keep the passages clear. However, strong or persistent coughing can become an irritant. Repeated coughing causes your bronchi to narrow, which can irritate the interior walls of the breathing passages.

Causes of persistent cough

Persistent coughing is frequently a symptom of a viral infection in the upper respiratory tract, which includes your nose, sinuses and airways. Colds and flu (influenza) are common examples of this kind of infection. Your voice box may become inflamed from the infection (laryngitis), causing pain and hoarseness.

Coughing also results from throat irritation caused by the drainage of mucus down the back of your throat, a condition known as postnasal drainage. Coughing may also occur with various chronic disorders.

People with allergies and asthma often have bouts of involuntary coughing, as do people who smoke. Many irritants in the environment, such as smog, dust and secondhand smoke, as well as meteorological conditions, such as cold or dry air, can produce coughing.

Sometimes coughing is caused by stomach acid that backs up into your esophagus or, in rare cases, your lungs. This condition is called gastro-esophageal reflux. Some people may develop a "habit" cough, which can often occur despite the lack of any underlying condition. Persistent cough can also be a side effect of certain medications.

Medical help

Short-lived (acute) bronchitis usually disappears in a matter of days. Contact a doctor if you experience shortness of breath or a fever of 101 F or higher for more than three days. If your cough lasts for more than 10 days with no end in sight, seek medical attention.

Home remedies

Take these steps to help relieve a persistent cough:

Drink plenty of fluids
Fluids help keep your throat clear. Drink water or fruit juices — not soda or coffee.

Use a humidifier
The air in your home can get very dry, especially during the winter. Dry air irritates your throat when you have a cold. Using a humidifier to moisturize the air will make breathing easier.

Suck on hard candy or lozenges
Hard candy or medicated throat lozenges may help soothe simple throat irritation and prevent coughing if your throat is dry or sore.

Try honey
Drink a cup of warm tea or warm lemon water that is sweetened with honey. Mix 2 teaspoons of honey with the warm liquid.

A study of children age 2 and older found honey at bedtime seemed to reduce nighttime coughing and improve sleep.

Due to the risk of infant botulism, a rare but serious form of food poisoning, never give honey to a child younger than age 1.

Elevate your bed
Sleep with the head of your bed elevated. Raise your bed 4 to 6 inches if your cough is caused by a backup of stomach acid. Also avoid food and drink within two to three hours of bedtime.

Avoid cough syrups
Don't waste your money on over-the-counter cough medicines because they aren't effective. See page 43.

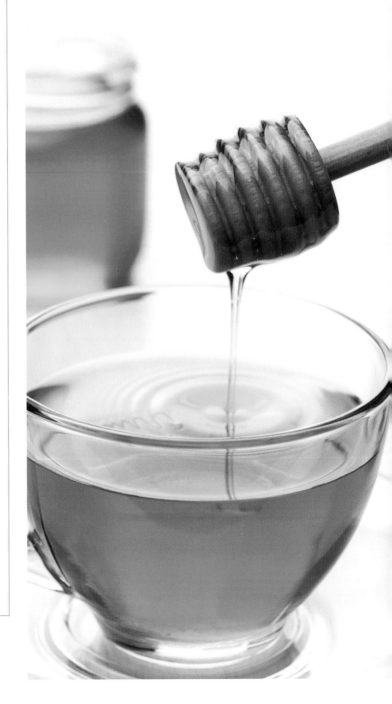

Cramps and charley horses

A cramp, sometimes called a charley horse, is actually a muscle spasm — a sudden, involuntary contraction of one or more muscles into a painful knot. Overuse or strain of a muscle, dehydration, or simply holding a single position for a prolonged period may result in the muscle cramp.

Almost everyone gets a cramp at some point in the course of day-to-day activities. For example, people who become fatigued and dehydrated while participating in sports in warm weather often complain of muscle cramps.

Writer's cramp affecting the thumb and first two fingers of your writing hand results from using the same muscles to grip a pen or pencil for long periods. At home, you can develop cramps in your hand or arm after spending long hours using a paintbrush or garden tool.

A common type of cramp— nocturnal cramps — occurs in your calf muscles or toes during sleep. The cause of this type of cramp is unknown but frequency seems to increase with age.

Medical help

Muscle cramps usually disappear on their own, and are rarely serious enough to require medical care. However, if you experience frequent and severe muscle cramps or if your cramps disturb your sleep, see your doctor.

Home remedies

If you have a muscle cramp, these actions may provide relief:
- Gently stretch and massage a cramping muscle.
- For lower leg (calf) cramps, put your weight on the leg and bend your knee slightly.
- For upper leg (hamstring) cramps, straighten your legs and lean forward at your waist. Steady yourself with a chair.
- Apply heat to relax tense, tight muscles.
- Apply cold to sore or tender muscles.
- Drink plenty of water. Fluid helps your muscles function normally.

Prevention
To prevent muscle cramps:
- Stretch your leg muscles daily, using the stretches for the Achilles tendon and calf as shown on page 97.
- Stretch your muscles carefully and gradually warm up before participating in vigorous activity.
- Stop exercising as soon as a cramp begins.
- Drink plenty of liquids every day. Fluids help your muscles contract and relax and keep muscle cells hydrated and less irritable. Drink fluids before any exercise activity.

Croup

Croup, marked by a harsh, repetitive cough, is a viral infection that develops most often in young children. The cough is similar to the noise of a seal barking, which can be frightening for both the children and their parents.

The harsh sounds of coughing are the result of swelling around the vocal cords and windpipe (trachea). When the cough reflex forces air through this narrowed passage, the vocal cords vibrate with the barking sound. Because children have smaller air passages, those younger than age 5 are more susceptible to the symptoms of croup.

In addition to the coughing, a child with croup may have difficulty breathing in. The child may become agitated and begin crying — actions that make inhaling even more difficult.

Croup typically lasts five or six days. During this time, symptoms may fluctuate back and forth between mild and severe. Symptoms are usually worse at night.

Medical help

Seek immediate medical attention if your child:
- Makes noisy, high-pitched breathing sounds when inhaling
- Begins drooling or has difficulty swallowing
- Seems agitated or extremely irritable
- Struggles to breathe
- Has a fever of 103.5 F or higher

Call 911 or your local emergency number for help if the child is in severe distress, unresponsive, blue or dusky.

Home remedies

Keep your child comfortable when he or she has croup with a few simple measures:
- *Stay calm.* Comfort or distract your child — cuddle, read a book or play a quiet game. Crying only makes breathing more difficult.
- *Moisten the air.* Use a cool-air humidifier in your child's bedroom or have your child breathe warm, moist air in a steamy bathroom. Researchers have questioned the benefits of humidity as part of emergency treatment for croup, but moist air seems to help children breathe easier — especially when croup is mild.
- *Get cool.* Sometimes breathing fresh, cool air helps. If it's cool outdoors, wrap your child in a blanket and walk outside for a few minutes.
- *Hold your child in an upright position.* Sitting upright can make breathing easier. Hold your child on your lap, or place your child in a favorite chair or infant seat.
- *Offer fluids.* For babies, water, breast milk or formula is fine. For older children, warm soup or frozen fruit pops may be soothing.
- *Encourage your child to rest.* Sleep can help your child fight infection.

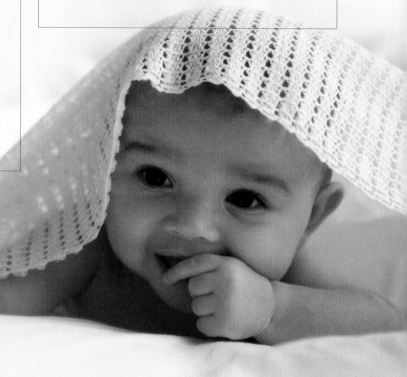

Cut and scrapes

Everyday cuts and wounds often don't require a trip to the emergency room. Yet proper care is essential to avoid infection and other complications. The guidelines on page 52 can help you in caring for simple wounds.

What about puncture wounds?

A puncture wound doesn't usually result in excessive bleeding. Often, in fact, little blood flows, and the wound seems to close quickly. This doesn't mean that treatment is unnecessary. You may require medical attention.

A puncture wound — such as from stepping on a nail, tack, wood splinter or glass — may be dangerous because of the risk of infection. The object that caused the puncture may carry spores of tetanus or other bacteria, especially if the object has been exposed to dirt. For shallow wounds, follow the self-care steps and advice on seeking medical help. A puncture wound may need to be cleaned by a doctor.

What about scarring?

No matter how you treat cuts, all wounds that penetrate deeper than the first, or outermost, layer of skin will form a scar when healed. Even small, superficial wounds can change skin tone or form a scar if infection or re-injury occurs. Following the guidelines on page 52 may help minimize these complications.

When a healing wound is exposed to sunlight, it can darken permanently. This darkening can be prevented by covering the area with clothing or sunblock with a sun protection factor (SPF) over 30 whenever you're outside during the first six months after the injury occurred.

A scar usually thickens about two months into the healing process. Within six months to a year, the scar tissue thins out.

Scar tissue that continues to enlarge or thicken is called a keloid. Surgical incisions, vaccinations, burns or even a scratch can cause keloids. The tendency to develop keloids is often inherited, and the darker the skin, the greater the likelihood of this happening.

When was your last tetanus shot?

A cut, laceration, bite or other wound that penetrates the skin, even if minor, can lead to a tetanus infection. Tetanus is a serious bacterial disease caused by a toxin that leads to muscle stiffness, especially of the jaw muscles. Tetanus is sometimes called lockjaw.

Immunization is vital. The tetanus vaccine usually is given to children as part of the diphtheria, tetanus and acellular pertussis (DTaP) vaccine. Adults generally need a tetanus booster every 10 years.

If a wound is deep and dirty, your doctor may recommend an additional booster even if your last one was within 10 years. Boosters should be given within two days of the injury.

Medical help

If bleeding persists — if blood spurts or continues to flow after several minutes of direct pressure — emergency care is necessary. Are stitches needed? A deep, gaping or jagged-edged wound with exposed fat or muscle will require stitches to hold it together. Was this an animal or human bite? Seek medical care.

Home remedies

If you plan to treat a wound, it's important to wash your hands with soap and water or an alcohol-based hand sanitizer beforehand to help avoid infection or other complications. The following guidelines can help you care for simple wounds:

Stop the bleeding
Minor cuts and scrapes usually stop bleeding on their own. If not, apply gentle pressure with a clean cloth or bandage.

Keep the wound clean
Rinse the wound with clear water. Clean the area around the wound with soap and a washcloth (but don't scrub the wound itself). Keep soap out of the wound, as it can cause irritation.

If dirt or debris remains in the wound after washing, use tweezers cleaned with alcohol to remove the particles. If debris still remains embedded in the wound, don't attempt to remove it by yourself — contact your doctor.

Thorough wound cleaning reduces the risk of infection and tetanus. There's no need to use hydrogen peroxide, iodine or an iodine-containing cleanser, which can be irritating to injured tissue.

Consider the source
Puncture wounds or other deep cuts, animal bites, or particularly dirty wounds put you at higher risk of infections, including tetanus. If the wound is serious, you may require antibiotics or an additional tetanus booster (see page 51).

Prevent infection
After cleaning the wound, if desired, you can apply a thin layer of petroleum jelly or an antibiotic ointment, such as Neosporin or Polysporin. These products don't make the wound heal faster, but they can discourage infection and allow the wound to close more efficiently. Certain ingredients in some ointments may cause a mild rash in some people. If a rash appears, stop using the ointment.

Cover the wound
Exposure to air will speed healing, but bandages can help keep the wound clean, keep harmful bacteria out and protect the wound from additional irritation. Blisters that are opened and draining are vulnerable to infection and should be covered until a scab forms.

Change the dressing
Change the bandage at least once a day or whenever it becomes wet or dirty to help prevent infection. If you're allergic to tape adhesive, switch to sterile gauze and paper tape or pressure netting. These supplies generally are available at pharmacies and drug stores.

Dandruff

Dandruff is a chronic scalp condition, marked by intensive itching and flaking skin on your scalp. Although dandruff isn't contagious and is rarely serious, it can be embarrassing.

The causes of dandruff are many, including dry skin, irritated and oily skin (seborrheic dermatitis), psoriasis, eczema, a yeastlike fungus called malassezia, not shampooing often enough or thoroughly enough, and scalp sensitivity to hair care products (contact dermatitis).

Babies get dandruff, too

A type of dandruff called cradle cap can affect babies. This disorder, which causes a scaling, crusty scalp, is most common in newborns, but it can occur anytime during infancy. Although it can be alarming for parents, cradle cap isn't dangerous and usually clears up on its own by the time a baby is a year old. To treat cradle cap:
- Gently rub your baby's scalp with your fingers or a rough washcloth to loosen the scales.
- Wash your baby's hair once a day with mild baby shampoo.
- If the scales don't loosen easily, rub petroleum jelly or a few drops of mineral oil onto your baby's scalp. Let it soak into the scales for a few minutes, and then brush and shampoo your baby's hair as usual. If you leave the oil in your baby's hair, the scales may accumulate and worsen the cradle cap.

Medical help

If dandruff persists or your scalp becomes irritated or severely itchy, you may need a prescription shampoo, or you may have some other skin condition. See your doctor.

Home remedies

To treat dandruff:
- *Shampoo regularly.* Start with a mild, nonmedicated shampoo. Gently massage your scalp to loosen flakes. Rinse thoroughly.
- *Use medicated shampoo for stubborn cases.* Look for shampoos containing pyrithione zinc, salicylic acid, coal tar or selenium sulfide in brands such as Head & Shoulders, Neutrogena T/Sal or T/Gel, Denorex or Selsun Blue. The medicated shampoo Nizoral A-D is intended to kill dandruff-causing fungi that live on your scalp. This shampoo is available over-the-counter or by prescription. Try rotating between two types of these shampoos.
- *If you use tar-based shampoos, use them carefully.* These products can leave a brownish stain on light-colored or gray hair and make the scalp more sensitive to sunlight.
- *Cut back on styling products.* Hair sprays, styling gels, mousses and hair waxes can all build up on your hair and scalp, making them oilier.
- *Eat a healthy diet.* A diet that provides enough zinc, B vitamins and certain types of fats may help prevent dandruff.
- *Get a little sun.* Sunlight may be good for dandruff. But because exposure to ultraviolet light damages your skin and increases your risk of skin cancer, don't sunbathe. Instead, just spend a little time outdoors. And be sure to wear sunscreen on your face and body.
- *Try tea tree oil.* This herbal product seems to reduce dandruff. The oil comes from the leaves of the Australian tea tree and has been used for centuries as an antiseptic, antibiotic and antifungal agent. It's now included in some shampoos found in natural foods stores. The oil may cause allergic reactions in some people.

Depression

Almost everyone feels down from time to time — a period of several days or a week in which you seem to be in a funk. This feeling usually goes away, and you're able to regain your normal outlook on life.

Having "the blues" isn't the same as having depression. Depression is a chronic illness that can lead to a variety of serious emotional and physical problems. Rather than being something you can simply "snap out of," depression typically requires long-term treatment, involving medications and psychological counseling.

If you're depressed, you may find little, if any, joy in life. You may have no energy, feel unworthy or guilty for no reason, find it difficult to concentrate, and become irritable. You might wake up after only a few hours of sleep or experience changes in your appetite — eating either too little or too much. You may experience a sense of hopelessness and deep anxiety, or even feel as if life isn't worth living.

Medical help

If depressive symptoms last more than a few weeks, or if you're feeling hopeless or suicidal, it's important to seek help. For many people, the most effective treatment is a combination of therapies. Contact your family doctor or ask for a referral to a psychiatrist, who is trained as a medical doctor and can help you find out if a medical illness might be contributing to your symptoms. If your symptoms are mild but persistent, a psychologist may be helpful. Psychologists are trained in psychotherapy, which is effective in treating both depression and anxiety.

Is it depression?

Signs of major depression	Signs of feeling down (minor depression)
• Persistent lack of energy • Lasting sadness • Irritability and mood swings • Recurring sense of hopelessness • Continual negative view of the world and of others • Overeating or loss of appetite • Feelings of unworthiness or guilt • Inability to concentrate • Recurrent early-mornng awakening or other changes in sleep patterns • Inability to enjoy pleasurable activities • Feeling as if you'd be better off dead	• Feeling down for several days but still able to function normally in daily activities • Occasional lack of energy, or a mild change in sleeping patterns • Ability to enjoy some recreational activities • Stable weight • Quickly passing sense of hopelessness

Home remedies

To help ease depression, try these tips:

- *Share your feelings.* Talk to a trusted friend, partner, family member or spiritual counselor. He or she can offer support, guidance and perspective.
- *Spend time with other people.* Social interaction generally is good, but make sure to spend your time with positive people, not those who may make your symptoms worse.
- *Do things you enjoy.* Engage in activities that have interested you in the past, but also don't be afraid to try something new.
- *Exercise regularly.* Physical activity can reduce the symptoms of depression. Consider walking, jogging, swimming, gardening or taking on active projects that you enjoy.
- *Avoid alcohol and illicit drugs.* It may seem like alcohol or drugs lessen symptoms of depression, but in the long run they generally make them worse and make your condition that much harder to treat.
- *Get plenty of sleep.* A good night's sleep is especially important when you're depressed. If you're having trouble sleeping, talk to your doctor about what you can do.
- *Don't take on too much responsibility all at once.* If you have large tasks, divide them into smaller ones. Set simple goals you can accomplish.
- *Look for opportunities to be helpful.* You feel better about yourself when you can help others, even in a small way.

St. John's wort

Studies suggest that St. John's wort may be beneficial in treating mild to moderate depression, but not major depression. The greatest concern with using this herb is the potential for serious interactions with other medications. Check with your doctor before taking this herb if you take prescription medications, as harmful interactions are possible.

SAMe

SAMe occurs naturally in the human body, and a synthetic version of the compound is a popular dietary supplement in the United States. Studies indicate SAMe may be effective for treating depression in some individuals.

Omega-3 fatty acids

Eating a diet rich in omega-3s or taking omega-3 supplements may help ease depression, along with providing other health benefits. These healthy fats are found in certain foods, such as cold-water fish, flaxseed, flax oil and walnuts.

Relaxation therapies

A number of relaxation therapies may help relieve some symptoms of depression by helping you deal with stress and anxiety — conditions that can heighten depression. These therapies include massage, yoga, meditation, relaxed breathing, and self-expression through music and art.

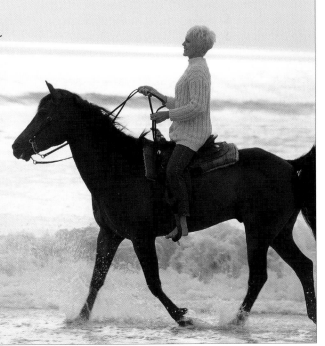

Diabetes

Diabetes (diabetes mellitus) is a disease that affects the way your body uses blood sugar (blood glucose) — which is your body's main source of energy.

Your body breaks down the food you eat and converts it into glucose, which is absorbed into the bloodstream. Insulin, which is made by the pancreas, helps move the glucose from the bloodstream into your cells, where it's burned for energy. If you have diabetes, your body produces little or no insulin. Or the insulin doesn't work very well, so too much glucose remains in your blood.

The most common forms of diabetes are known as type 1 and type 2. Other forms include gestational diabetes, which can occur during pregnancy.

Type 1 vs. type 2

Type 1 diabetes is an autoimmune disease. Your own immune system attacks your pancreas, destroying cells, so little if any insulin is made. Without insulin to help move glucose into your cells, glucose stays in your bloodstream. Daily insulin shots are needed. The disease most often develops when you're young, although adults also can develop type 1 diabetes.

Type 2 diabetes is by far the most common form of the disease. Your pancreas may make some insulin, but your cells become resistant to it, so too much glucose stays in your bloodstream. Being overweight makes it harder for your body to use insulin. Type 2 diabetes usually develops in adults, but as more children and teens become overweight, the incidence of type 2 diabetes is increasing.

What's prediabetes?

Prediabetes means that your blood glucose level is higher than normal but not high enough for you to be diagnosed with type 2 diabetes. Long-term damage associated with diabetes — especially to your heart and blood vessels — may already be starting if you have prediabetes.

But you can prevent or delay type 2 diabetes by making healthy changes to your lifestyle. In a major study on diabetes prevention, those in the lifestyle-treatment group (who ate a healthy diet and engaged in moderately intense physical activity) cut their risk of diabetes in half.

Diabetes warning signs

Often, prediabetes has no signs or symptoms, so it's important to know your blood glucose level. Watch for two classic warning signs of diabetes:
- Excessive thirst
- Frequent urination

Other signs and symptoms may include:
- Constant hunger
- Unexplained weight loss
- Weight gain (more common in type 2)
- Flu-like symptoms, including weakness and fatigue
- Blurred vision
- Slow-healing cuts or sores
- Tingling or loss of feeling in the hands and feet
- Recurring infections of gums and skin
- Recurring vaginal or bladder infections

Medical help

Diabetes requires expert care. If you think you may have diabetes, see your doctor. Also see a doctor if you have diabetes and your symptoms seem to be worsening.

Home remedies

If you want to play an active role in your health, take control of your diabetes with these steps.

Exercise

Regular physical activity and exercise is essential to lowering your blood glucose level and improving your body's ability to use insulin or other diabetes medications. Getting plenty of exercise may even reduce the amount of diabetes medication you need to take.

You can become more physically active in many small ways, such as taking the stairs instead of the elevator. Learn how to avoid blood glucose problems while exercising. Before you start a fitness program, discuss precautions you may need to take with your doctor.

Research has shown that a sedentary lifestyle is a major contributing factor in diabetes. If your lifestyle requires you to sit at a desk most of the day, look at ways to get on your feet. Request a standing desk, stand and stretch frequently, take regular trips to get a drink of water — even these minor actions help.

Monitor your blood sugar

Good management of your blood glucose level is key to feeling your best and preventing the complications of diabetes. Knowing how often and when to test your blood glucose will depend on which type of diabetes you have and on your treatment plan. If you have type 1 diabetes and take insulin, test your blood glucose at least twice a day. Your doctor may advise testing more often.

If you have type 2 diabetes and don't need insulin, test your blood glucose as often as needed to be sure it's under control. This can mean daily testing or twice a week. Discuss the schedule with your doctor.

Eat healthy foods

Follow these basic tips:

- *Stick to a schedule.* Eat three meals a day. Be consistent in the amount of food you eat and the timing of your meals. If you're hungry after dinner, choose a food low in calories or carbohydrates before going to bed, such as raw vegetables.
- *Focus on fiber.* Eat a variety of fresh fruits, vegetables, legumes and whole-grain foods. These high-fiber foods help control blood glucose and are low in fat and rich sources of vitamins and minerals.
- *Limit foods that are high in saturated and trans fat.* Choose lean cuts of meat and use low-fat or fat-free dairy products. Use small amounts of healthy oils and trans fat-free spreads instead of shortening and butter.
- *Choose proteins low in saturated fat.* If you eat too much protein, your body stores the extra calories as fat. Choose fish and poultry more often than red meat.
- *Eat fewer sweets.* Candy, cookies and other sweets aren't forbidden, but they're often high in fat and calories. Count them in your total carbohydrate intake.

Lose weight

Being overweight is by far the greatest risk factor for type 2 diabetes. If you're overweight, losing even a few pounds can improve your blood glucose level.

Home remedies

Diabetes and your feet

Good foot care is essential if you have diabetes. Diabetes can impair blood flow to your feet and cause severe nerve damage. Left untreated, minor foot injuries can quickly develop into open sores (ulcers) that may be difficult to treat — even leading to tissue death (gangrene). Put your best foot forward with these simple foot care tips:

- *Wash your feet daily.* Wash in lukewarm water once a day. Dry them gently, especially between the toes. Sprinkle talcum powder or cornstarch between your toes to keep the skin dry. Use a moisturizing cream or lotion on the tops and bottoms of your feet to keep the skin supple and soft.

- *Inspect your feet daily.* Check your feet for blisters, cuts, sores, redness or swelling once a day. If you have trouble bending over, use a hand mirror to inspect the bottoms of your feet, or ask someone to help you.

- *Trim your toenails carefully.* Trim your nails straight across. If you have any nail problems or numbness in your feet, ask your doctor about professional nail trimming.

- *Don't go barefoot.* Protect your feet from injury with comfortable socks and shoes, even indoors. Make sure new shoes fit well, too. Even a single blister can lead to an infection that won't heal.

- *Wear clean, dry socks.* Wear socks made of fibers that pull (wick) sweat away from your skin, such as cotton and special acrylic fibers — not nylon. Avoid socks with tight elastic bands that reduce circulation or that are thick or bulky. Bulky socks often fit poorly, and a poor fit can irritate your skin.

- *Use foot products cautiously.* Don't use a file or scissors on calluses, corns or bunions. You can injure your feet that way. Also, don't put chemicals on your feet, such as wart removers. See your doctor or foot specialist (podiatrist) for problem calluses, corns, bunions or warts.

- *Don't smoke or use other types of tobacco.* Smoking reduces blood flow to your feet. Talk to your doctor about ways to quit smoking or to stop using other types of tobacco.

- *Schedule regular foot checkups.* Your doctor can inspect your feet for early signs of nerve damage, poor circulation or other foot problems. You may be referred to a podiatrist.

- *Take foot injuries seriously.* Contact your doctor if you have a sore or other foot problem that doesn't begin to heal within a few days. Your doctor may prescribe antibiotics to treat infection. In other cases, infected tissue may be drained or removed. Sometimes, surgery is needed to remove infected bone or increase blood flow to the affected area.

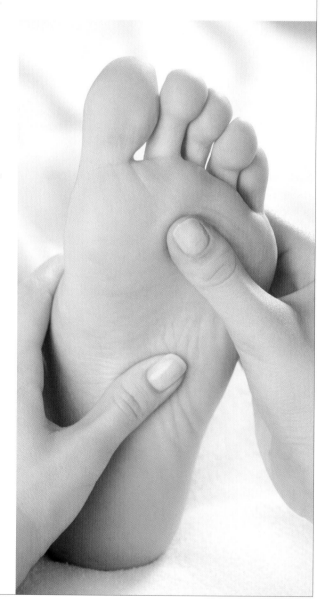

Diaper rash

Diaper rash causes reddish, puffy, irritated skin in the diaper area. The rash generally is caused by a combination of moisture, acid in urine or stool, and chafing of diaper fabric on your baby's skin. Some babies also get a rash from the detergent used to launder cloth diapers, or from plastic pants, elastic, or certain types of disposable diapers and wipes. Sometimes a yeast infection may be the cause of a rash.

Diaper rash may alarm parents and irritate babies, but most occurrences can be resolved with simple at-home treatments.

Cloth or disposable diapers?

Many parents wonder about which kind of diaper to use for their babies. When it comes to preventing diaper rash, there's no compelling evidence that cloth diapers are better than disposable ones or vice versa, although disposables may keep baby's skin slightly drier. Because there's no clear-cut "best" diaper, use whatever works best for you and your baby. If one brand of disposable diaper seems to irritate your baby's skin, try out another brand.

Medical help

See your doctor if the tips at right don't help, if the rash is crusty, blistered or weepy, or if your baby has a fever.

Home remedies

To treat or prevent diaper rash:

- *Change your baby's diapers frequently.* This helps to minimize the exposure of sensitive skin to urine and stool.
- *If using cloth diapers, use softened water for washing and rinsing.* Make sure that all the detergent is rinsed out.
- *Wash and pat the skin dry at each diaper change.* Use plain water or a mild soap and water.
- *Apply a thin barrier of cream or ointment.* Various diaper rash medications are available without a prescription. Talk to your doctor or pharmacist for specific recommendations. Some popular over-the-counter creams, including Balmex and Desitin, contain zinc oxide as the active ingredient. These products are usually applied in a thin layer to the irritated region throughout the day to soothe and protect the skin. Zinc oxide products can also be used on healthy skin to prevent diaper rash.
- *Allow your child to go without a diaper for short periods of time.* Exposing skin to air is a natural and gentle way to let it dry. To avoid messy accidents, try laying your baby on a large towel and engage in some playtime while he or she is bare bottomed.
- *Experiment with brands.* Try switching to a different brand if you use disposable diapers.
- *Avoid diaper wipes.* Many contain irritating perfumes and alcohol. Use a washcloth with plain water instead.

Diarrhea

Diarrhea is loose, watery stools, often accompanied by abdominal cramps. You also may notice abdominal pain and other flu-like signs and symptoms, such as low-grade fever, achy or cramping muscles, and headache.

Diarrhea may be acute or chronic. Acute diarrhea is something that nearly everyone experiences at some time, and it usually clears up within days. The most common cause of acute diarrhea is a viral infection of the digestive tract. Bacteria and parasites also can cause diarrhea, sometimes with bloody stools and high fever. Infection-induced diarrhea can be extremely contagious. Nausea and vomiting may precede it. Diarrhea also can be a side effect of many medications, particularly antibiotics.

Chronic diarrhea generally lasts longer than four weeks and may signal a serious underlying medical problem such as chronic infection, inflammatory bowel disease, irritable bowel syndrome (IBS), microscopic colitis or certain kinds of cancer.

Diarrhea also can be a sign of lactose intolerance or from the use of products made with artificial sweeteners, such as sorbitol and mannitol. In these cases, the diarrhea usually improves with a change in diet.

Medical help

Contact your doctor if diarrhea persists for more than a week, or if you become dehydrated or see traces of blood in your stool or in the toilet bowl. Also seek medical attention if you have severe abdominal or rectal pain, a temperature of more than 101 F, or signs of dehydration despite drinking fluids. Your doctor may prescribe antibiotics for diarrhea caused by some bacteria and parasites. However, not all bacterial diarrhea requires treatment with antibiotics, and antibiotics don't help viral diarrhea.

Home remedies

Diarrhea caused by infections typically clears on its own without medications. Over-the-counter anti-diarrheal products, such as Imodium A-D, Pepto-Bismol and Kaopectate, may slow bowel movements, but they won't speed recovery. Focus your attention on preventing dehydration and easing the symptoms of diarrhea as you recover:

- Drink plenty of clear liquids, including water, clear sodas (caffeine-free), broths and weak tea.
- Add semisolid and low-fiber foods gradually as your bowel movements return to normal. Try soda crackers, toast, eggs, rice or chicken.
- Avoid eating dairy products, fatty foods or highly seasoned foods for a few days.
- Avoid caffeine, alcohol and nicotine.

Probiotics

Probiotics can help maintain a proper microorganic balance in your intestinal tract. Food sources of probiotics include yogurt, miso, tempeh, and some juices and soy drinks. Probiotic supplements may help manage diarrhea, especially after treatment with antibiotics.

Diarrhea in infants

Diarrhea in infants should be closely monitored. Contact your doctor if diarrhea persists for more than 12 hours and if your child:

- Hasn't had a wet diaper in eight hours
- Has a temperature of more than 102 F
- Has bloody stools
- Has a dry mouth or cries without tears
- Is unusually sleepy, drowsy or unresponsive

Dizziness

Lightheadedness, weakness, loss of balance, faintness, wooziness and unsteadiness on your feet are signs and symptoms associated with dizziness. You may feel that you or your surroundings are rotating — a condition known as vertigo. You may need to support yourself or hold on to something to maintain your balance.

Dizziness is one of the most common reasons why people visit their doctors. Although it may be disabling, dizziness rarely signals a serious, life-threatening condition. Treatment depends on the cause and on your symptoms, but it's usually effective.

Fainting is a sudden, brief loss of consciousness that may accompany dizziness. Fainting may be caused by a variety of medical disorders, including heart disease, severe coughing spells and circulatory problems. It may also be related to:

- Blood pressure and heart rhythm medications
- Excessive sweating, vomiting or diarrhea causing fluid loss
- Upsetting news or sights
- Rapid drop in blood pressure, for example, when you stand quickly from a sitting or reclining position

Medical help

Seek medical care if symptoms of dizziness persist for weeks or become severe. Seek emergency care for fainting or when dizziness is accompanied by signs and symptoms such as pain in the chest or head, trouble with breathing, numbness or continuing weakness or paralysis, irregular heartbeat, confusion, decreased responsiveness, memory loss, seizure, trouble talking, problems with vision or coordination, blood in stools (sometimes indicated by black tarry stools) or other signs of blood loss, or nausea or vomiting.

Home remedies

If you feel faint or dizzy, find a safe place to lie down or sit down. If you lie down, elevate your legs slightly to return blood to your heart. If you can't lie down, then sit leaning forward and put your head between your knees.

Prevention of dizziness

- *Stand and change positions slowly.* Do this particularly when turning from side to side or when changing from lying down to standing up. Before standing up in the morning, sit on the edge of the bed for a minute or two.
- *Pace yourself.* Take breaks when you are active in heat and humidity.
- *Dress appropriate to weather conditions This will help you to avoid overheating.*
- *Drink enough fluids to avoid dehydration.* Aim to drink at least 48 to 64 ounces a day, unless your doctor tells you to limit fluids.
- *Avoid caffeine and alcohol.* Excessive use of these substances can contribute to dehydration and worsen signs and symptoms of dizziness.
- *Use caution.* Don't drive a car or operate dangerous equipment if you feel dizzy.
- *Check your medications.* Your doctor may need to adjust your prescriptions.

Dry eyes

Healthy eyes are continuously covered by a thin layer of fluid — a tear film that remains stable between the blinks of your eyelids. The tear film lubricates the eyes and helps maintain clear vision.

Dry eyes occur when the tear film is destabilized, often due to decreased fluid production from your tear glands. This allows dry spots to form on the surface of your eyes. Poor tear quality also can cause dry eyes.

Dry eyes are a common source of discomfort. The condition usually affects both eyes, especially in women after menopause. Some drugs — such as antihistamines, sleep medications and some high blood pressure medications — also can cause dry eyes or make them worse.

Signs and symptoms of dry eyes may include:
- Stinging, burning or scratchy sensations
- Stringy mucus in or around your eyes
- Increased eye irritation from smoke or wind
- Eye fatigue after short periods of reading
- Sensitivity to light
- Difficulty wearing contact lenses
- Tearing
- Blurred vision, often worsening at the end of the day

Medical help

Seek medical care if the condition continues despite self-care efforts. Your doctor may prescribe a medication for chronic dry eyes or refer you to a specialist if needed.

Home remedies

To help reduce dryness in your eyes:
- *Try over-the-counter artificial tears.* Choose a type that doesn't contain a redness remover (these may worsen symptoms). If you're sensitive to preservatives, try single-use preservative-free lubricants. If your eyes are dry overnight, use a gel-type lubricant at bedtime. Ask your doctor which option might work best for you.
- *Avoid air blowing in your eyes.* Don't direct hair dryers, car heaters, air conditioners or fans toward your eyes.
- *Blink often.* Consciously blinking repeatedly helps spread your tears more evenly across the surface of your eyes.
- *Avoid rubbing your eyes.*
- *Cover your eyes.* Wear glasses on windy days and goggles while swimming or skiing.
- *Add moisture to the air.* In winter, a humidifier can improve the dry indoor air. Some people use specially designed glasses that form a moisture chamber around the eye, creating additional humidity.
- *Don't smoke and avoid secondhand smoke.* Avoid all types of smoke, even the type from a fireplace or burning leaves.

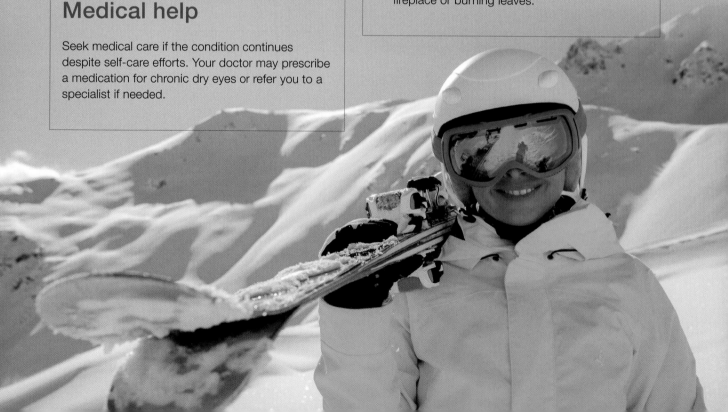

Dry mouth

Saliva is a clear liquid mixture that moistens your mouth and helps with digestion. It's produced in your salivary glands. When there's a lack of saliva, your mouth feels dry and the saliva seems thick and stringy. Your lips crack, and splits in the skin appear at the corners of your mouth. A sore throat may develop, and you may have difficulty speaking and swallowing.

Dry mouth may seem like little more than a nuisance, but it can have a very negative impact on your enjoyment of food and the health of your teeth. The medical term for dry mouth is xerostomia.

Without enough saliva, the food in your mouth will seem dry and difficult to swallow. You won't be able to taste properly because of a dry tongue. And your digestion will be affected. Dry mouth can also contribute to tooth decay, since saliva limits the growth of bacteria and washes away food and plaque.

Although the treatment of dry mouth depends on the cause, it's often a side effect of medication. Dry mouth is also more common as you age.

Medical help

If you've noticed persistent signs and symptoms of dry mouth, make an appointment with your family doctor or your dentist.

Home remedies

If the cause of dry mouth either can't be determined or can't be resolved, the following tips may help improve your symptoms and keep your teeth healthy:

- *Encourage salivation.* Chewing sugar-free gum or sucking on sugar-free hard candies helps stimulate saliva production.
- *Limit your caffeine intake.* Caffeine can make your mouth drier.
- *Avoid sugary or acidic foods and candies.* They increase the risk of tooth decay.
- *Brush with a fluoride toothpaste.* Ask your dentist if you might benefit from prescription fluoride toothpaste.
- *Include other fluoride products.* Use a fluoride rinse or brush-on fluoride gel before bedtime.
- *Don't use a mouthwash that contains alcohol because this can make your mouth drier.*
- *Stop all tobacco use.*
- *Sip water regularly.*
- *Try over-the-counter saliva substitutes.* Look for ones containing carboxymethyl cellulose or hydroxyethyl cellulose, such as Biotene Oralbalance.
- *Avoid using over-the-counter antihistamines and decongestants.* These medications can make symptoms worse.
- *Breathe through your nose, not your mouth.*
- *Add moisture to the air.* Use a room humidifier at night.

Dry skin

Dry skin is often a temporary or seasonal problem — one that you experience only in winter or summer, for example — but the problem may remain a lifelong concern. Patches of itchy, irritated skin announce its arrival.

Although your skin is often driest on your arms, lower legs and sides of your abdomen, the locations where these dry patches form can vary considerably from one person to the next.

Signs and symptoms of the condition will depend on your age, health status, living environment, the amount of time you spend outdoors, and the specific cause of your problem.

With dry skin, you may have one or more of the following:

- Sensation of skin tightness, especially after showering, bathing or swimming
- Skin that appears shrunken or dehydrated
- Skin that feels and looks rough rather than smooth
- Itching that sometimes may be intense
- Slight to severe flaking, scaling or peeling skin
- Fine lines or cracks in the skin
- Redness

Causes

Dry skin is caused primarily by your amount of exposure to certain environments, particularly when the air is dry and has low humidity. Common causes of dry skin include:

- **Weather.** In general, your skin is driest in the winter, when temperatures and humidity levels plummet. Winter conditions also tend to make many existing skin conditions worse. But the reverse may be true if you live in desert regions, where temperatures can soar but humidity levels remain low.
- **Interior heating and air conditioning.** Central heating and cooling systems, as well as wood-burning stoves, space heaters and fireplaces, all reduce humidity and dry your skin.
- **Hot baths and showers.** Frequent cleaning and rinsing, especially if you like hot water and long soaks, breaks down the lipid barriers in your skin and dries you out. So does

frequent swimming, particularly in chlorinated pools.

- **Harsh soaps and detergents.** Many popular soaps and detergents strip lipids and water from your skin. Deodorants and antibacterial soaps are usually the most damaging, as are many shampoos, which dry out your scalp.
- **Sun exposure.** Like any type of heat, the sun dries your skin. Yet damage from ultraviolet (UV) radiation penetrates far below the top layer of skin. The most significant damage occurs deep, where collagen and elastin fibers break down much more quickly than they should, leading to deep wrinkles and loose, sagging skin (solar elastosis). Sun-damaged skin may have the appearance of dry skin.

Medical help

Most cases of dry skin respond well to lifestyle changes and home remedies. See your doctor if:

- Your skin doesn't improve in spite of your best efforts
- Dry skin is accompanied by redness
- Dryness and itching interfere with sleeping
- You have open sores or infections from scratching
- You have large areas of scaling or peeling skin
- The itching is out of proportion to the dry skin

Home remedies

Consider this: It's more important to prevent moisture from leaving your skin than it is to try adding moisture back into your skin. Although it may not be possible to achieve flawless skin, the following measures can help keep it moist and healthy:

Moisturize your skin

Moisturizers form a seal over your skin that helps keep water from evaporating from its surface. Thicker moisturizers work best, such as the over-the-counter brands CeraVe, Eucerin and Cetaphil. Also consider using cosmetics that contain moisturizers. If your skin is extremely dry, you may want to apply an oil, such as baby oil, while your skin is still moist. Oil has more staying power on the skin than moisturizers do.

Avoid harsh, drying soaps

If you have dry skin, it's best to use cleansing creams, gentle skin cleansers, and bath or shower gels with added moisturizers. Choose mild soaps that have added oils and fats, such as Neutrogena, Basis or Dove. Avoid deodorant and antibacterial detergents, which are especially harsh. You might want to experiment with several brands until you find one that works well for you. Your skin should feel soft and smooth after cleansing, never tight or dry. If your skin is particularly dry, you may want to apply soap only to body folds, such as your underarms and groin.

Limit bath time

Hot water and long showers or baths remove oils from your skin. Limit your bath or shower time to about 10 minutes or less, and use warm, rather than hot, water.

Moisturize after bathing

After washing or bathing, gently pat or blot your skin dry with a towel so that some moisture remains on the skin. Immediately moisturize your skin with an oil or cream to help trap water in the surface cells.

Use a humidifier

Hot, dry indoor air can parch sensitive skin and worsen itching and flaking. A portable home humidifier or one attached to your furnace adds moisture to the air inside your home. Choose a humidifier that meets your budget and special needs. Be sure to keep the humidifier clean to ward off bacteria and fungi growth.

Choose natural fabrics

Natural fibers such as cotton and silk allow your skin to breathe. Wool, although it certainly qualifies as natural, can irritate even normal skin. When you wash your clothes, try to use detergents without dyes or perfumes.

Suppress itching

If dry skin causes itching, apply cool compresses to the area. To reduce inflammation, use a nonprescription hydrocortisone cream or ointment, containing at least 1 percent hydrocortisone. Limit application to less than a week.

Ear infection

A middle ear infection (otitis media) is one of the most common conditions of early childhood. Studies show that 3 out of 4 children have had at least one middle ear infection by age 3. Many have multiple episodes. Though less common, adults also can get ear infections.

The condition often starts with a respiratory infection, such as a cold, which is caused by a virus. Colds may cause swelling and inflammation in the narrow passageway (eustachian tube) that connects the middle ear to the nose. Inflammation may block one of the tubes completely, trapping fluid in the middle ear and causing infection.

Signs and symptoms include earache, feeling of blockage in the ear, fever of 100 F or higher, and temporary hearing loss. Children may tug or pull at their ears, cry more than usual, have trouble sleeping, and be unusually irritable. A discharge may drain from the ear.

Your doctor will examine your child and study the symptoms. Many cases of ear infection won't need treatment such as antibiotics. The next steps depend on many factors, including your child's age and medical history.

Before prescribing antibiotics, many doctors may recommend a wait-and-see approach for the first 72 hours, especially if the child has few symptoms. Most ear infections cause discomfort and worry but generally clear up on their own in just a few days.

Some doctors believe people who have a middle ear infection with discharge should also be given antibiotics. However, it's not universally agreed that the antibiotics are necessary or will work to prevent the infection.

If the medication is effective, your child should start feeling better in a few days. Be sure to take the antibiotic for the full length of the prescription. Remember, antibiotics won't help an infection caused by a virus — and the overuse of antibiotics contributes to strains of bacteria that resist the medications.

What about recurrent infections?

Many ear infections resolve on their own after about three days. However, some long-lasting or recurrent ear infections may lead to complications. Usually, fluid buildup from an ear infection disappears in a few weeks. But sometimes it remains in the middle ear for months, which can damage the eardrum and bones of the middle ear, causing long-term hearing loss.

Medical help

Contact your child's doctor if pain lasts more than a day or so or it's associated with fever. About 80 percent of children's ear infections resolve on their own, without using antibiotics. But antibiotics may be used if your child is under 2 years old, has recurrent middle ear infections or has a high-risk medical condition. Keep immunizations up to date: Some may help reduce the risk of middle ear infections.

Home remedies

To find relief from ear infections, try the following:

- *Over-the-counter medications.* If your child is uncomfortable, ask the doctor about using an over-the-counter pain reliever such as acetaminophen (Tylenol, others) or ibuprofen (Advil, Motrin IB, others). Use the correct dose for your child's age and weight. Don't give aspirin to children, due to the risk of Reye's syndrome — a rare but serious condition. Giving over-the-counter cough or cold medications also isn't recommended for children age 2 and younger.
- *Warm compress.* It may help to place a warm, moist cloth over the affected ear.
- *Distractions.* When caring for your child, plan low-key activities, such as reading books aloud, singing or playing board games. And don't underestimate the benefits of some extra cuddling.

Can you prevent ear infections?

Preventing ear infections is difficult, but these approaches may help reduce your child's risk:

- Breast-feeding has been shown to reduce the frequency of ear infections and should be considered, if possible.
- When bottle-feeding, hold your baby in an upright position.
- Avoid exposing your child to tobacco smoke.
- Keep immunizations up to date. Certain vaccines, such as the pneumoccal vaccine, can reduce the risk of middle ear infections in your child.

Do children outgrow ear infections?

For many parents, coping with the ear infections of their young children is almost as routine as changing wet diapers. But most children stop having ear infections by age 4 or 5. As your child matures, the eustachian tubes become wider and more angled, making it harder for inflammation to block the passageway and easier for fluid to drain out of the ear. Although ear infections still may occur in adults, they probably won't develop as often.

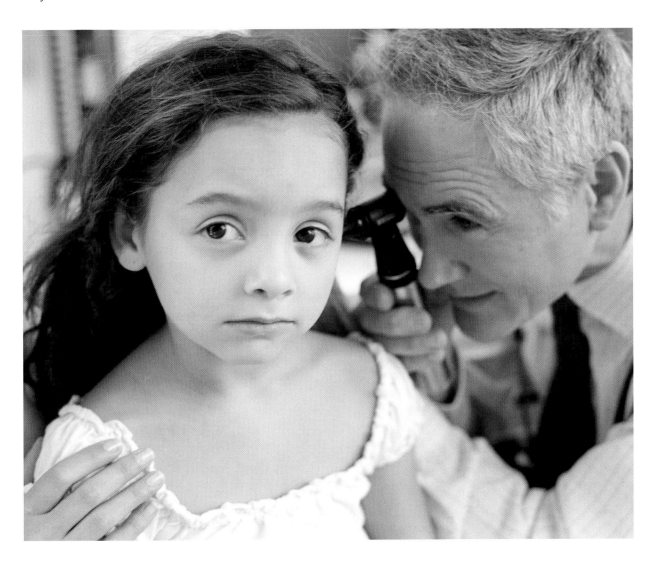

Ear ringing

Some people may hear a persistent ringing or buzzing sound in their ears when no other sounds are present. The noise, known as tinnitus, seems to originate in their heads and not come from their surroundings.

Although bothersome, tinnitus usually isn't a sign of something seriously wrong. The cause of the sound is often unknown. Sometimes, however, tinnitus may be treated if an underlying cause can be identified: Earwax buildup or a foreign object in the ear canal or infection. The sound also may be caused by high doses of aspirin or large amounts of caffeine.

Persistent ringing in one or both ears may also be a symptom of a more serious ear disorder, particularly if it's accompanied by hearing loss or dizziness.

Medical help

If ringing in your ear gets worse, persists or is accompanied by hearing loss or dizziness, consider getting a full evaluation from your doctor. The doctor may pursue further testing. Although most causes of tinnitus are benign and not life-threatening, it can be a difficult and frustrating condition to treat.

Home remedies

Strategies to help you cope with a persistent ringing or buzzing sound in your ear include:

- *Explore aspirin alternatives.* If aspirin in high doses has been recommended to you, ask your doctor about alternatives. If you're taking aspirin on your own, try lower doses or another kind of over-the-counter pain medication.
- *Avoid nicotine, caffeine and alcohol.* All of these substances may aggravate the condition.
- *Manage stress.* Stress can make tinnitus worse. Stress management, whether through relaxation therapy, biofeedback or exercise, may provide some relief.
- *Limit causes.* Try to determine a cause for the tinnitus, such as exposure to loud noise, and avoid the cause, if possible.
- *Protect your ears.* Wear earplugs or some form of hearing protection when you're exposed to loud noise, such as when you're working with yard equipment (snow blower, leaf blower, lawn mower or power tools).
- *Cover your symptoms.* Some people benefit from covering up the ringing sound with another, more acceptable sound, such as soft music from a radio as you fall asleep.
- *Try a masker.* Some people may benefit by wearing a device that fits in the ear and produces white noise that masks the ringing.

Earwax blockage

Earwax is part of your body's natural defenses. It helps protect the ear canal by trapping dirt and slowing the growth of bacteria. At times, though, blockage of the ear canal occurs if you produce too much earwax or a buildup of earwax becomes too hard to wash away naturally. This may give you an earache or feeling of fullness in the affected ear, or cause ear noise (tinnitus).

Note of caution

The safest way to have earwax removed is to have it done by your doctor. Your ear canal and eardrum are extremely delicate structures that can be damaged easily. Don't poke them with objects such as cotton swabs, paper clips or bobby pins, especially if you have had ear surgery, have a hole in your eardrum, or are having ear pain or drainage. These objects may push the wax deeper, damaging the ear canal lining and eardrum.

Flushing wax out of the ears should be avoided if you've had an eardrum perforation or ear surgery, unless your doctor approves. If infection is a concern, don't flush your ears.

Some people use ear candling, a technique that involves placing a lighted, hollow, cone-shaped candle into the ear, to remove earwax. This procedure doesn't work and may cause additional injury, such as burns or perforations.

Home remedies

If you think you may have earwax blockage — and your eardrum doesn't contain a tube or have a hole (perforation) in it — this procedure may help you remove excess earwax:

1. Soften the earwax by applying a few drops of baby oil, mineral oil or glycerin with an eyedropper twice a day, for no more than four to five days.
2. When the wax is softened, fill a bowl with water heated to body temperature. If the water is colder or hotter, it may make you feel dizzy during the procedure.
3. With your head upright, grasp the top of your ear and pull upward. With your other hand, squirt the water gently into your ear canal with a 3-ounce rubber-bulb syringe. Then, tilt your head and drain the water into the bowl or sink.
4. You may need to repeat this process several times before the extra wax falls out.
5. Gently dry your outer ear with a towel or a hand-held hair dryer.

Earwax removal kits sold in stores can be effective. If you're unsure which one is right for you, ask your doctor.

Medical help

Many people have difficulty washing wax out of their ears, even after following the procedure described at right. Asking your doctor to remove earwax may seem unnecessary, but it can help relieve the blocked sensation in the ear. Your doctor can remove the excess wax safely and effectively using a similar procedure.

Eczema

The terms *eczema* and *dermatitis* are both used to describe inflammation of the skin. The condition occurs in many forms but usually involves patches of dry, swollen, reddened and itchy skin. Patches may thicken and develop blisters or weeping sores in severe cases.

The skin inflammation can make you feel uncomfortable and self-conscious, but it's generally not life-threatening or contagious.

Contact dermatitis results from the direct contact of skin with an irritant, which includes poison ivy, rubber, metals, jewelry, perfume and cosmetics.

Neurodermatitis can occur when something such as a tight garment rubs or scratches (or causes you to scratch) your skin, resulting in a chronic itch-scratch-itch cycle.

Seborrheic dermatitis (known as cradle cap in infants) appears on the scalp and face as itchy dandruff or areas of greasy scales.

Stasis dermatitis may cause the skin at your ankles to discolor, thicken and itch. This condition can lead to infection.

Atopic dermatitis causes itchy, thickened, cracking skin, most often in the folds of the elbows or backs of the knees. It frequently runs in families and is often associated with seasonal allergies and asthma.

Medical help

See your doctor if:
- You're so uncomfortable that you're losing sleep or distracted from your daily routines
- Your skin is painful
- You suspect your skin is infected
- You've tried self-care steps without success

Home remedies

To relieve symptoms of eczema and prevent the condition from worsening:

- *Try to identify and avoid triggers.* Irritants may include rapid changes of temperature, sweating and stress. Some people should avoid direct contact with wool products, such as rugs, bedding and clothes, as well as harsh soaps and detergents.
- *Apply an anti-itch cream or calamine lotion to the affected area.* A nonprescription hydrocortisone cream, containing at least 1 percent hydrocortisone, can temporarily relieve itching. A nonprescription oral antihistamine (Benadryl, others), may be helpful if the itching is severe.
- *Avoid scratching whenever possible.* Cover the itchy area if you can't keep from scratching it. Trim nails and wear gloves at night.
- *Apply cool, wet compresses.* Covering the area with bandages and dressings can help protect the skin and prevent scratching.
- *Take a warm bath.* Sprinkle the bath water with baking soda, uncooked oatmeal or colloidal oatmeal — a finely ground oatmeal made for the bathtub (Aveeno, others). Or add 1/2 cup of bleach to a 40 gallon bathtub filled with warm water. The diluted bleach bath is thought to kill bacteria that grow on the skin.
- *Choose mild soaps without dyes or perfumes.* Be sure to rinse the soap completely off your body.
- *Moisturize your skin.* Use a non-perfumed oil or cream to seal in moisture while your skin is still damp from a bath or shower. If your skin is already dry, consider using a lubricating cream.
- *Use a humidifier.* Hot, dry indoor air can parch sensitive skin and worsen itching and flaking. A portable home humidifier or one attached to your furnace adds moisture to the air inside your home.
- *Wear cool, smooth-textured cotton clothing.* Avoid clothing that's rough, tight, scratchy or made from wool.

Elbow pain

Most elbow pain results from overuse injuries, often from activities requiring repetitive hand, wrist or arm movements.

- Bursitis and tendinitis are common sources of pain in your elbow. Bursitis may produce a small, egg-shaped, fluid-filled sac at the tip of your elbow. Keep pressure off the elbow, such as using a soft foam elbow pad.
- Dislocated elbow occurs when the ends of the joint bones are forced from their natural positions. Dislocation is very painful and limits movement.
- Hyperextended elbow occurs when your elbow is pushed beyond its normal range of motion, often as a result of a fall or misplay during the swing of a racket or bat.
- Tennis elbow and golfer's elbow are two similar conditions. Tennis elbow affects the tendons on the outer side of your elbow, while golfer's elbow affects tendons on the inner side. Common causes include swinging a racket or club, pitching a baseball, painting, using a screwdriver or hammer, raking, typing, or any movement requiring twisting arm motions or repetitive gripping.

Medical help

If the pain hasn't improved in a day or two, see your doctor.

Seek medical care immediately if:

- Your elbow seems deformed, or dislocated
- The area around your elbow is very sensitive to pressure
- Your arm or hand becomes numb
- Your elbow is very stiff and has limited range of motion after a fall
- The pain in your arm is severe
- Your elbow is hot and inflamed and you have a fever.

Home remedies

If pain and swelling occurs in your elbow and in the tissues beneath your elbow, try these tips:

- *Practice P.R.I.C.E.* (see page 157). Support your elbow with a splint or sling for a few days then begin to move it through as complete a range of motion as possible. Elbows have a tendency to stiffen after injury, so movement is the best prevention.
- *Take an anti-inflammatory medication.* Commonly options include ibuprofen (Advil, Motrin IB, others) and acetaminophen (Tylenol, others). However, seek medical advice if you have any kidney problems or stomach problems before using NSAIDs.

Pain prevention while participating in sports

- *Use good technique.* Ask a trainer to review your technique to see if you're using the proper mechanics.
- *Warm up.* Prepare for repetitive work-related tasks by participating in fitness and strengthening routines. Gently stretch the forearm muscles before and after use.
- *Get in shape.* Prepare for any sport with appropriate preseason conditioning. Do strengthening exercises with a hand weight by flexing and extending the wrists.
- *Try support bands.* Wear forearm support bands just below your elbow.
- *Heat up.* Try applying a warm pack for five minutes before activity and an ice pack after heavy use.
- *Lift properly.* When lifting anything — including free weights — keep your wrist rigid and stable to reduce the force transmitted to your elbow. Lift only the amount of weight that is comfortable, as straining to lift excess weight can lead to injury.

Enlarged prostate gland

The prostate is a walnut-sized gland in males, tucked beneath the bladder, which produces semen. Testosterone, the male sex hormone, causes the prostate to enlarge as men get older.

As the prostate enlarges, some men develop bothersome urinary symptoms. Untreated prostate gland enlargement can block the flow of urine out of the bladder and can cause bladder, urinary tract or kidney problems.

Signs and symptoms of an enlarged prostate gland (benign prostatic hyperplasia, or BPH) may include a weak or slow urine stream, trouble starting urination, stopping and starting during urination, dribbling at the end of urination, frequent and sometimes urgent need to urinate, frequent nighttime urination, and not being able to completely empty the bladder.

Having an enlarged prostate doesn't necessarily mean your symptoms will get worse. Only about half the men with prostate gland enlargement have symptoms that become noticeable or bothersome enough for them to seek medical treatment. In some men, symptoms eventually stabilize and may even improve over time.

Medical help

If you're having urinary problems, it's best to see your doctor for an evaluation. If your symptoms aren't too burdensome, self-care measures may be all you need. If self-care measures don't work, you may benefit from prescription medications that shrink the prostate gland or improve urine flow. Surgery can reduce the size of the prostate.

Home remedies

Lifestyle changes can often help control the symptoms of an enlarged prostate and prevent your condition from getting worse.

- *Avoid drinking fluids an hour or two before bedtime.*
- *Limit your intake of caffeine and alcohol.*
- *When you first feel the urge to urinate, go.* Waiting too long may damage your bladder muscle.
- *Schedule bathroom visits.* Try to urinate regularly during the day, such as every four to six hours.
- *Keep moving.* Even a small amount of physical activity can help reduce urinary problems caused by an enlarged prostate.
- *Limit decongestants or antihistamines.* These drugs tighten the band of muscles around your urethra that controls urine flow, which makes it harder to urinate.
- *Consider saw palmetto.* In some men, this herb may be an effective treatment for managing mild to moderate symptoms. (However, some studies have not found the herb to be effective.) Because saw palmetto is generally safe, it doesn't hurt to give it a try.

Eye scratch

The most common types of eye injury involve the cornea — the clear, protective dome of tissue that covers the iris and pupil at the front of the eye. The cornea can be scratched when it comes in contact with dirt, sand, wood shavings, metal particles or even the edge of a piece of paper.

Usually the scratch is superficial, and this is called a corneal abrasion. Everyday activities may lead to abrasions, for example, getting a wood chip caught in your eye while doing home repairs, or being scratched by a child who accidentally brushes your cornea with a fingernail.

Because the cornea is extremely sensitive, an abrasion can be painful. A scratched cornea might make you feel like you have sand and grit in your eye. You may also have tears, blurred vision, light sensitivity, and redness in and around the eye.

Some corneal abrasions become infected and result in a corneal ulcer, which is a serious problem. Abrasions that are caused by plant matter, such as a pine needle, can cause a delayed inflammation that develops inside the eye.

Medical help

In case of any injury to the eye, seek prompt medical attention.

Home remedies

Immediate steps you may take to treat a corneal abrasion include:

- *Rinse your eye with clean water (use a saline solution, if available).* You can use an eyecup or small, clean drinking glass positioned with its rim resting on the bone at the base of your eye socket. If your work site has an eye-rinse station, use it. Rinsing the eye may wash out a foreign object.
- *Blink several times.* This movement may remove small particles of dust or sand.
- *Pull the upper eyelid over the lower eyelid.* The lashes of your lower eyelid can brush a foreign object from the undersurface of your upper eyelid.
- *Don't rub your eye after an injury.* Touching or pressing on your eye can worsen a corneal abrasion.
- *Don't touch your eyeball with cotton swabs, tweezers or other instruments.* This can aggravate the abrasion.
- *Don't try to remove an object that's embedded in your eyeball.* Avoid trying to remove a large object that makes closing the eyelid difficult.

Eyestrain

Eyestrain occurs when your eyes tire from intense use, such as driving a car or reading for extended periods, exposure to bright lights or glare, or spending long hours in front of a computer monitor. Signs and symptoms may include:

- Sore, tired or burning eyes
- Watery or dry eyes
- Blurred or double vision
- Headache
- Sore neck
- Increased sensitivity to light

Although eyestrain is often fatiguing and annoying, it usually isn't serious. Typically, the strain goes away once you're able to rest your eyes. In some cases, the signs and symptoms of eyestrain indicate an underlying eye condition that needs treatment.

Using a computer for long periods of time is one of the most common causes of eyestrain. Although you may not be able to change the nature of your job or avoid all the factors that cause eyestrain, you can take steps to reduce its effects.

Medical help

If self-care doesn't relieve your eyestrain symptoms, see your eye doctor if you have ongoing symptoms that include:

- Eye discomfort
- Noticeable change in vision
- Double vision

Home remedies

Simple adjustments in how you read, work or surf the Internet may help give your eyes a much-needed rest.

- *Direct your light.* For close-up work, use light that's directed on what you're doing. When reading, position the light source behind you and direct the light onto the page. When reading at a desk, use a shaded light positioned in front of you.
- *Take frequent eye breaks throughout the day.* Try to stand up and move around at least once every hour or so.
- *Blink often.* This helps to refresh and lubricate your eyes. Because many people blink less than normal when working at a computer, dry eyes often result from prolonged computer use.
- *Consider using artificial teardrops.* These over-the-counter products can help relieve dry eyes from prolonged computer work. Lubricating drops that don't contain preservatives may be used as often as you need. If the drops contain preservatives, don't use them more than four times a day. Avoid eyedrops with a redness remover, as these ingredients may worsen dry eye symptoms.

Tips for computer work

- Make sure your work space is set up in an eye-friendly way.
- Position your monitor directly in front of you about 20 to 28 inches from your eyes.
- Check the lighting and reduce glare. Bright lighting and too much glare can make it difficult to see objects on your screen.
- Place your keyboard directly in front of your monitor, not at an angle.
- Get proper computer eyewear.

Eye sty

A sty is a red, painful lump that forms on the outer edge of your eyelid — although sometimes it can form on the inner surface of the eyelid. A sty may resemble a boil or pimple. Usually the lump is filled with pus, develops gradually over several days, and ruptures in about a week.

The cause of a sty is bacterial infection, usually from staphylococcus, or "staph." Due to the swelling, it may become difficult to see clearly because you can't fully open your eye.

More than one sty can occur at a time, leading to a widespread inflammation of your eyelid — a condition known as blepharitis. Fortunately, most sties disappear on their own after a few days. In the meantime, you may be able to relieve the pain and discomfort with simple self-care treatments.

Medical help

Most sties are harmless to your eye. Still, you should see your doctor if a sty causes one of the following problems:

- Interferes with your vision
- Recurs frequently with successive infections
- Doesn't disappear on its own
- Doesn't respond to self-care
- Develops redness or swelling that extends beyond the lid into your face or cheek

Home remedies

Until the sty goes away on its own, self-care usually involves:

- Leaving the sty alone. Don't try to pop the sty or squeeze the pus from the sty.
- Applying a clean, warm compress four times a day for 10 minutes to help encourage the sty to burst. Once the sty has ruptured, rinse your eye thoroughly and keep the area clean.

Prevention
To prevent recurrent infections:

- *Wash your hands.* Practice good hand-washing techniques and keep your hands away from your eyes. If you have children, make sure they practice proper hand-washing techniques because they may be more prone to sties.
- *Take care with cosmetics.* You can help prevent recurrent infections by not using old cosmetics or sharing makeup with anyone.
- *Make sure your contact lenses are clean.* If you wear contact lenses, follow your doctor's advice on disinfecting your lenses and wash your hands thoroughly before inserting your contacts.

Fatigue

Almost everyone experiences fatigue at some time. After a long weekend of yard work or a hectic day with the children, it's natural to feel tired and worn out. This kind of physical and emotional fatigue is normal. You can usually restore your energy with a little rest or exercise.

If you feel tired all the time, or if exhaustion becomes overwhelming, you may worry that your condition is more serious than just being worn out. In some cases, fatigue is a symptom of an underlying condition that may require medical treatment.

Most of the time, however, fatigue can be traced to one or more of your daily habits or routines. Chances are you know what's causing your fatigue. And with a few lifestyle changes, it's likely that you'll find the resources to revitalize your life.

Fatigue isn't the same thing as sleepiness, although you often have a desire to sleep. Nor is it a lack of motivation. Fatigue can result from physical or emotional factors. Physical fatigue usually strengthens later in the day, while emotional fatigue often improves as the day progresses.

Common causes of physical fatigue

- Poor eating habits
- Lack of sleep
- Being out of shape
- Over-the-counter drugs, such as pain relievers, cough and cold medicines, antihistamines and allergy remedies
- Prescription drugs, such as tranquilizers, muscle relaxants, sedatives and blood pressure medications
- Dehydration
- Warm interior environments

Medical causes of fatigue

Fatigue may also be an early symptom of the following medical conditions:
- Low red blood cell count
- Cancer
- Low thyroid activity
- Diabetes
- Various acute or chronic infections
- Alcoholism
- Heart disease
- Rheumatoid arthritis
- Sleep disorder
- Electrolyte imbalance (when the blood levels of minerals, such as sodium and potassium, are too high or too low)

Many of these illnesses are accompanied by other signs and symptoms, such as muscle aches, pain, nausea, weight loss, sensitivity to cold and shortness of breath.

What is chronic fatigue syndrome?

Chronic fatigue syndrome is a complicated disorder characterized by extreme fatigue that may worsen with physical or mental activity, but doesn't improve with rest. Besides fatigue, symptoms include memory loss, sore throat, joint or muscle pain, painful lymph glands, abdominal pain or bloating, headaches and unrefreshing sleep.

Although there are many theories about what causes the condition, in most cases the cause is unknown. There's no specific treatment for chronic fatigue syndrome. In general, doctors aim to simply relieve signs and symptoms.See your doctor.

Medical help

If fatigue persists even after you've had ample rest and the fatigue lasts for two weeks or longer, you may have a problem that requires medical care. See your doctor.

Home remedies

Before discussing concerns with your doctor, consider the possibility that your fatigue may be resolved with one or more of these lifestyle changes:

- *Get an adequate night's sleep.* Aim for seven to eight hours of uninterrupted sleep.
- *Follow a sleep schedule.* Regularly go to bed and wake up at about the same time each day.
- *Give yourself time to relax.* Ask others for help if you're feeling overworked or overwhelmed.
- *Organize your daily schedule.* Prioritize the most important activities. Don't try to do everything.
- *Identify the factors that cause stress.* And then try to reduce your stress level.
- *Include more physical activity and exercise in your day.* Exercise gives you more energy. Increase activity gradually, especially if you've recently been inactive. If you're over age 40, it might be a good idea to consult your doctor before beginning a vigorous exercise program.
- *Increase daily exposure to fresh air at home and at work.* Fresh air gives you more energy.
- *Eat a balanced diet.* Include plenty of fruits, vegetables and whole grains. Steer clear of high-fat foods. Eat a healthy breakfast and don't skip other meals.
- *Create a plan to lose weight if you're overweight.* But avoid very low calorie diets that don't provide enough nutrients and increase fatigue.
- *Drink plenty of water.* If your urine is clear or pale yellow, you're probably getting enough fluid. If it's dark yellow, you probably need to drink more.
- *Review your medications.* This includes both over-the-counter and prescription drugs. Fatigue may be a side effect.
- *Quit smoking.* Smoking increases fatigue.
- *Reduce or eliminate the use of substances such as alcohol and caffeine.* These substances are known to affect sleep or cause fatigue.

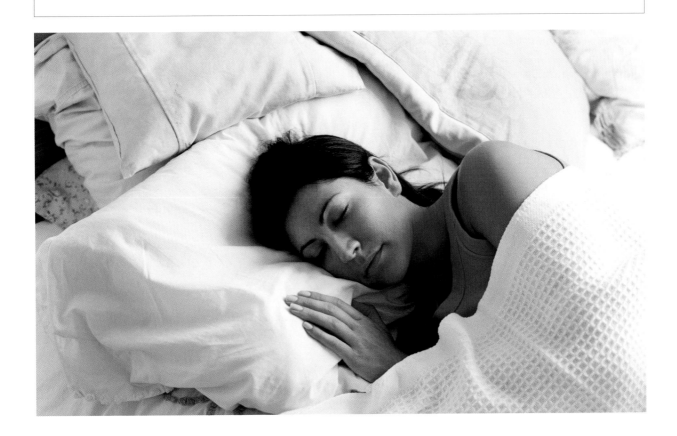

Fever

Even when you're well, your body temperature varies, and that variation is normal. In the morning your temperature is generally a little lower, and in the afternoon it's somewhat higher. The average healthy body temperature is around 98.6 F (37 C).

Temperatures under 100.4 F (38 C) are still considered normal. If they are 100.4 F or higher, it's often considered a fever.

Fever signals that something out of the ordinary is going on inside your body. It's not necessarily an illness, but it may be a sign of one. Fever may be accompanied by other symptoms, such as sweating, shivering, headache, muscle ache and weakness.

Most likely, when you have a fever, you're fighting a bacterial or viral infection. Rarely, it's the sign of a reaction — either to a medicine or to an inflammatory condition. Sometimes, it's difficult to identify the cause of fever.

Don't automatically try to lower your temperature if you have a fever. Over-the-counter medications may help, but sometimes it's better to leave it untreated. Fever seems to play a role in helping your body fight off infections. And lowering your temperature may mask other symptoms, making it harder to identify the cause. Usually fever goes away within a few days.

Fever in children

Signs of fever in small children include irritability, disinterest and inability to feed or sleep well. Children under age 6 may have a sudden change in temperature accompanied by a seizure (febrile seizure). Although alarming, the seizure typically lasts less than five minutes and has no lasting effects.

If a seizure happens, lay your child on his or her side. Don't put anything in the mouth or try to stop the convulsions. Call 911 or emergency medical help if it's the first febrile seizure or it lasts more than five minutes.

Sometimes a low-grade fever accompanies teething or a recent immunization. Fever with ear pulling may indicate a middle ear infection.

If you're concerned, don't hesitate to call your doctor or other health care provider.

If medication is needed, it's usually provided in liquid form. For a small child, use a syringe (without a needle) to gently squirt the medicine in the back corners of the child's mouth.

Children and aspirin

Don't give aspirin to anyoneunder 18 years old, unless specifically recommended by the child's doctor. Rarely, aspirin causes a serious or even fatal disease called Reye's syndrome if given to children during a viral infection.

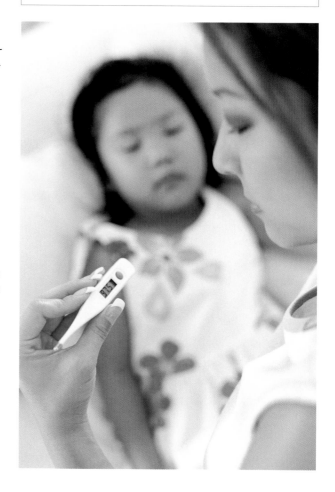

Medical help

Call your doctor in the following situations, especially if accompanied by a cough that produces phlegm, side pain, reddened skin, painful urination, or diarrhea:

- Temperature of more than 104 F (40 C)
- Temperature of more than 102 F (38.9 C) for 48 hours or more
- Fever over 100.4 F (38 C) for more than three days or one that returns after it was gone for 24 hours

A fever is only one sign of illness, and older adults or anyone with lowered immunity may run a fever when ill. Inform your doctor of any contagious diseases that people around you have had, including flu, colds, measles and mumps.

Call 911 or emergency medical help immediately if any of these occur in addition to fever:

- Severe headache or unusual eye sensitivity to bright light
- Severe swelling of the throat or difficulty breathing
- Significant stiff neck and pain when the head is bent forward, often paired with altered mental status, such as confusion
- Persistent vomiting
- Fast pulse, rapid breathing and lightheadedness when standing

Call 911 or emergency medical help if your baby has a fever along with a bulging soft spot on the head. Call your doctor immediately if your baby is 3 months old or younger with a rectal temperature of 100.4 F (38 C) or higher.

Home remedies

Here are steps you can take to make yourself or your child more comfortable during a fever:

Drink plenty of fluids
Fever can cause fluid loss and dehydration. Drink water, juices or rehydration drinks such as Pedialyte (for infants). A child may want to suck on frozen fruit pops. Pedialyte ice pops also are available.

Rest
Rest is necessary for recovery. By contrast, physical activity can raise your body temperature and, if moderately intense, sap some of your energy.

Take medication
Take acetaminophen (Tylenol, others) and ibuprofen (Advil, Motrin, others) according to label instructions or as recommended by your doctor. Don't use these medications at the same time or alternate doses unless you are instructed to do so by your doctor.

Avoid taking too much medication. High doses or long-term use of acetaminophen may cause liver or kidney damage, and acute overdoses can be fatal.

For temperatures below 102 F (38.9 C), don't use fever-lowering drugs unless advised by your doctor. Sometimes a low-grade fever helps the body eliminate a virus, such as a cold.

If you're not able to get your child's fever down, don't continue to give more medication. Call your doctor instead.

Soak in lukewarm water
Especially for fevers with high temperatures, a lukewarm five- to10-minute soak in the bathtub can be cooling. Giving a sponge bath to a small child has the same effect. If the sponge bath causes shivering, stop the bathing and dry your child. Shivering raises the body's internal temperature — shaking muscles generate heat.

Fibromyalgia

Fibromyalgia is a chronic condition characterized by widespread pain in your muscles, ligaments, tendons and soft tissue. But even after extensive tests, your doctor is unable to find anything specifically wrong with you.

The type of pain varies but is often described as a constant dull ache. Women are more likely to develop the disorder than are men. You're more likely to have it if a relative also has the condition. And it tends to develop in early or middle adulthood.

Signs and symptoms of fibromyalgia include:
- Widespread aching, lasting more than three months
- Fatigue and nonrestorative, nonrestful sleep
- Tender points — where slight pressure can cause pain — at multiple locations, usually where muscle is attached to bone
- Associated problems such as headaches, irritable bowel syndrome and pelvic pain

Signs and symptoms may vary depending on the weather, level of stress, physical activity or time of day. Many people awaken tired, even after sufficient sleep. Although people with fibromyalgia feel muscle pain, this is not a disease of the muscles.

The science of fibromyalgia is still emerging, but the condition may eventually be found to be a disorder of the nervous system. Medications used for this condition affect chemical receptors in the brain and spinal cord — they don't treat your muscles.

Depression or depressive feelings often accompany fibromyalgia and often require specific treatment. Similarly, stress usually worsens the symptoms of fibromyalgia.

Medical help

If you feel that you have excessive stress or depression from trying to cope with fibromyalgia, discuss your concerns with your doctor or a mental health provider.

Home remedies

Self-care and coping strategies are critical elements in the management of fibromyalgia.

Reduce stress

Develop a plan to avoid or limit overexertion and emotional stress. Allow yourself time each day to relax. But don't change your routine totally. People who quit work or drop all activity tend to do worse than those who remain active. Try stress management techniques, such as deep-breathing exercises or meditation.

Get enough sleep

Because fatigue is a common symptom of fibromyalgia, getting sufficient sleep is essential. Practice good sleep habits, such as going to bed in the evening and getting up in the morning at the same time each day. Try to limit daytime napping.

Exercise regularly

At first, exercise may increase pain, but doing it regularly often decreases symptoms. Appropriate exercises include walking, biking, swimming and water aerobics. Strengthen supportive muscles, especially abdominal muscles, to help improve your posture. Stretching and relaxation exercises also are helpful. A physical therapist can help you develop an exercise program.

Pace yourself

Develop a routine that alternates work with rest. Avoid long hours of repetitive activity. If you try to do too much on your good days, you may end up having more bad days.

Seek support

Find a support group that emphasizes maintaining health. Ask your family and friends for support.

Learn relaxation techniques

There are numerous therapies you can choose from. Most are low-risk techniques that may provide some benefits. Set aside time to practice them in your daily schedule. Relaxation techniques include:

- *Deep-breathing exercises.* Breathe in slowly and deeply through your nose to a count of five. Hold the air in your lungs for a count of five and then breathe out slowly through your mouth to a count of 10.
- *Progressive muscle relaxation.* Gently tighten and then relax muscle groups in your body one at a time, starting at either your head or your feet.
- *Meditation.* Focus on a single object or repeat a particular sound to help quiet your mind and relax your muscles.
- *Visualization.* Take an imaginary trip to a beautiful place. Use all of your senses to experience the location as fully as possible. Feel the sun's warmth and the gentle breeze. Listen to birds singing.

Flu

Influenza — commonly called the flu — is a viral infection that attacks your respiratory system, including your nose, throat, bronchial tubes and lungs.

If you're generally healthy and you catch influenza, you're likely to feel rotten for a few days, but you probably won't develop complications or need hospital care. If you have a weakened immune system or chronic illness, though, influenza can be fatal.

Initially, the flu may seem like a common cold with a runny nose, sneezing and sore throat (see page 43). But colds usually develop slowly, while the flu tends to strike suddenly. While a cold feels like a nuisance, you usually feel much worse with the flu. Signs and symptoms of the flu include:

- Fever
- Chills and sweats
- Headache
- Dry cough
- Muscular aches and pains, especially in your back, arms and legs
- Fatigue and weakness
- Nasal congestion
- Loss of appetite
- Diarrhea and vomiting in children

Flu viruses travel through the air in droplets when someone with the infection coughs, sneezes or talks. You can inhale the droplets directly, or you can pick up the germs by touching an object where the droplets have landed, such as a telephone or computer.

Not all flu is the same

The flu is caused by three types (strains) of viruses — influenza A, B and C. Type A can be responsible for the deadly influenza pandemics (worldwide epidemics) that strike every 10 to 40 years. Type B can lead to smaller, more localized outbreaks. Either type A or B can cause the flu that circulates almost every winter. Type C has never been connected with a large epidemic.

Medical help

If you have flu symptoms and are at risk of complications, see your doctor right away. Taking antiviral drugs within the first 48 hours after you first notice symptoms may reduce the length of your illness by a day or two and may help prevent more serious problems. Seek immediate medical care if you have signs and symptoms of pneumonia. These include a severe cough that brings up phlegm, a high fever and a sharp pain when you breathe deeply. If you have bacterial pneumonia, you'll need treatment with antibiotics.

Home remedies

If you do come down with the flu, these measures may help ease your symptoms:

- *Drink plenty of liquids.* Choose water, juice and warm soups to prevent dehydration. Drink enough so that your urine is clear or pale yellow.
- *Rest.* Get more sleep to strengthen your body and help your immune system fight against the infection.
- *Try chicken soup.* It's not just good for your soul — chicken soup really can relieve flu symptoms by helping to break up sinus congestion.
- *Consider pain relievers.* Use an over-the-counter pain reliever such as acetaminophen (Tylenol, others) or ibuprofen (Advil, Motrin, others) cautiously, as needed. Remember, pain relievers may make you feel more comfortable, but they won't make your symptoms go away any faster. They may also have side effects. For example, ibuprofen may cause stomach pain, bleeding and ulcers. If taken for a long period of time or in higher than recommended doses, acetaminophen can be toxic to your liver. Don't give aspirin to children or teens because of the risk of Reye's syndrome, a rare but potentially fatal disease.

Prevention

To reduce your risk of the flu:

- *Get an annual flu vaccination.* The best time to be vaccinated is October or November. This allows ample time for your body to develop antibodies to the flu virus before the peak flu season starts, which is typically between December and March in the Northern Hemisphere. However, getting a flu shot later is better than not getting one at all, and may still protect you. It takes up to two weeks to build immunity following a flu shot.
- *Wash your hands.* Thorough and frequent hand washing is the best way to prevent many common infections. Scrub your hands vigorously for at least 15 seconds, rinse well and turn off the faucet with a paper towel. Or use an alcohol-based hand gel containing at least 60 percent alcohol.
- *Eat right, sleep tight.* Both poor diet and poor sleep can lower your immunity and make you more vulnerable to infections. A balanced diet emphasizing fresh fruits and vegetables, whole grains, and small amounts of lean protein works best for most people. The amount of sleep needed for a healthy immune system varies. In general, adults seem to do best on seven to eight hours of sleep a night. Older children and teens need more rest — between nine and ten hours every night.

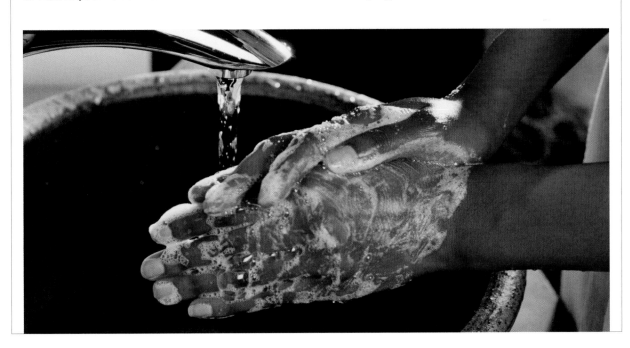

Foot and ankle pain

The foot is made up of 26 bones, 33 joints, and over a hundred muscles, tendons and ligaments. The ankle is the intricate, bony joint where the foot and leg meet. Given this complex structure and the amount of punishment that your feet and ankles have toendure every day, it's no wonder that pain can be so common. See also pages 96-97 regarding heel pain.

Sprains and strains

A sprain is an injury to a ligament — when the band of fibrous tissue connecting one bone to another in your joints is stretched or torn. The most common location for a sprain is in your ankle. A strain is an injury to a muscle or tendon — when the cord of tissue connecting muscle to bone is stretched or torn. See pages 131 and 156 for more.

Fractures

A stress fracture in the foot is really a hairline crack in the bone. It's often caused by the repetitive application of force, typically by overuse — such as repeatedly jumping up and down or running in high-impact activities such as basketball or track and field.

Achilles tendinitis

This is an inflammation of the Achilles tendon, which connects your calf muscles in the lower leg to your heel bone. It's often a running or other sports-related injury caused by overuse or intensive exercise, which strains the tendon. You'll feel a dull ache or pain, especially when you run or jump. The tendon may also be mildly swollen or tender.

Bunions

A bunion is an abnormal, bony bump that forms at the base of your big toe. The big toe joint becomes enlarged, forcing the toe to crowd against your other toes. The base of your big toe is pushed outward, extending beyond your foot's normal profile. Ill-fitting footwear or an inherited structural defect are often the cause of this condition. Shoe pressure over a bunion can be very painful and lead to callus formation. Arthritis of the big toe joint can develop as a result of bunion deformity.

Hammertoe and mallet toe

Unlike a bunion, hammertoe may occur in any toe (most commonly the second toe). The toe becomes bent, giving it a claw-like appearance, and may be painful. Hammertoe can result from wearing shoes that are too short, but also can occur in people with muscle and nerve damage from diseases such as diabetes. A mallet toe is a deformity in which the very end of the toe is bent downward.

Flatfeet

You have flatfeet when the arch on the inside of your foot is flattened, allowing your entire foot to touch the floor when you stand up. A common and usually painless condition, flatfeet may occur when the arches don't develop during childhood. It can also happen due to injury or from simple wear and tear. Flatfeet can become a problem if the condition forces your ankle to turn inward, throwing off the alignment of your leg.

Burning feet

Burning feet — the sensation that your feet are painfully hot – can be mild or severe. Burning feet can occur simply because your feet are tired. Infections, such as athlete's foot, also can cause-burning feet. The sensation can also develop as a result of damage to the nerves of the feet (peripheral neuropathy).

Does the shoe fit?

You can avoid many foot and ankle problems with shoes that fit properly. Here's what to look for:

- Adequate toe room — height, width and length. Avoid shoes with pointed toes.
- Low heels, which will help you avoid back problems.
- Laced shoes, which are roomier and more adjustable.
- Comfortable athletic shoes, strapped sandals or soft pumps with cushioned insoles. Avoid vinyl and plastic shoes. They don't breathe when your feet perspire, trapping moisture.

Buy shoes in the afternoon and evening. Your feet are smaller in the morning and swell throughout the day. Measure both feet. As you age, your shoe size (length and width) may change.

Medical help

Seek medical care immediately if:

- Your foot pain is severe and the area is swollen after an injury
- Your foot is hot and inflamed or you have a fever following the injury
- Your foot or ankle is deformed or bent in an abnormal position
- The pain is so severe that you can't move your foot
- You can't bear weight 72 hours after any injury

Home remedies

For foot and ankle pain
- Follow the instructions for P.R.I.C.E. (see page 157).

For a stress fracture
- Allow at least one month for healing. A cast or walking boot may be necessary, based on the location of the stress fracture.
- Avoid high-impact activities anywhere from six weeks to several months, based on stress fracture location and advice from your doctor.

For Achilles tendinitis
- Wear soft-soled running shoes, and avoid running or walking up or down hills.
- Avoid any impact on your heel for several days.
- Use gentle calf stretches daily (see page 311).

For bunions
- Wear shoes with adequate toe width that are made of soft leather.
- Have your shoes stretched in the area of the bunion.

- Wear sandals or lightweight shoes in the summer.
- Larger deformities may require special shoes.

For flatfeet
- Arch supports in well-fitting shoes may give you a better weight-bearing position.

For hammtertoe
- Special toe pads or cushions help protect the toe. Metatarsal pads may reduce pain in the ball of the foot behind the hammertoe. Stretching your shoes over the hammertoe to reduce pressure may be helpful.

For burning feet
- Wear nonirritating cotton or cotton-synthetic blend socks and shoes of natural materials that "breathe." A specially fitted insole also may help.
- Eliminate aggravating activities, such as standing for long periods.
- Bathe your feet in cool water.

Frostbite

Frostbite occurs when skin and underlying tissues freeze. The most common cause of frostbite is direct exposure to cold-weather conditions, but exposure to freezing materials, such as ice, also can cause frostbite. In subfreezing temperatures, the tiny blood vessels in your skin tighten, reducing the flow of blood and oxygen. Eventually, tissue cells are destroyed.

Frostbite can affect any part of your body. Your hands, feet, nose and ears are most susceptible because they are delicate and often exposed to cold.

Frostnip, the first stage of frostbite, irritates the skin but doesn't cause permanent damage. The first sign of frostnip may be a slightly painful, tingling sensation. With continued exposure, the skin becomes numb, feels hard and cold, and may turn deathly pale in color. Frostbitten areas, as they thaw, may burn with pain.

When frostbite is severe, the area will probably remain numb until it heals completely. Healing can take months, and the damage to your skin can permanently change your sense of touch.

Frostbite can damage deep layers of tissue. As deeper layers of tissue freeze, blisters may form. The blistering usually occurs over one to two days.

Medical help

Seek medical care if numbness remains during rewarming, you experience increased pain or discharge, you develop blisters, or damage to the skin appears severe.

Home remedies

Gradually warming the affected skin is the key to treating frostbite. To do so:

- *Protect your skin from further exposure.* If you're outside, warm your frostbitten hands by tucking them into your armpits. Protect your face, nose or ears by covering the area with dry, gloved hands. Don't rub the affected area and never rub snow on frostbitten skin.
- *Get out of the cold.* Once you're indoors, remove wet clothes.
- *Gradually warm frostbitten areas.* Put frostbitten hands or feet in warm water — 104 to 107.6 F (40 to 42 C). Wrap or cover other areas in a warm blanket. Don't use direct heat, such as a stove, heat lamp, fireplace or heating pad, because these can cause burns.
- *Don't walk on frostbitten feet or toes, if possible.* This will further damage the soft tissues on your feet.
- *If there's any chance the affected areas will freeze again, don't thaw them out.* If they're already thawed out, wrap them up so that they don't become frozen again.
- *Know what to expect as skin thaws.* If the skin turns red and there's a tingling and burning sensation as it warms, circulation is returning. But if numbness or sustained pain remains during warming or if blisters develop, seek medical attention.
- *Apply aloe vera gel or lotion to the affected area several times a day.* This helps reduce inflammation.

Gas, belching and bloating

Gas, belching and bloating are natural occurrences, typically caused by swallowed air in the gastrointestinal tract or by the normal breakdown of food during the digestive process. You may only occasionally experience these symptoms, or you may have to deal with them frequently or repeatedly in a single day.

Passing gas (flatulence)

Most intestinal gas (flatus) is produced in the colon. Gas buildup is typically caused by the fermentation of food, such as plant fiber. Gas can also form when your digestive system doesn't completely break down certain components in food, such as gluten or sugar. Other sources of gas may include changes in intestinal bacteria, medications and swallowed air.

Belching

Belching, or burping, is your body's way of getting rid of excess air from your stomach. You may swallow too much air if you eat or drink too fast, talk while you eat, drink carbonated beverages, or drink through a straw. Some people swallow air as a nervous habit. Indigestion and heartburn may be relieved by belching.

Bloating and gas pains

When gas is not expelled by belching or flatulence, it can build up in the stomach and intestines and lead to bloating. Abdominal pain, either mild and dull or sharp and intense, often occurs with bloating. Passing gas may relieve the pain. Bloating is also related to conditions such as irritable bowel syndrome or lactose intolerance.

In addition to eating fatty and gas-producing foods, such as beans and raw vegetables, bloating and gas pain may also result from stress and anxiety or from smoking.

Medical help

Bouts of excess gas, belching and bloating often resolve on their own. Consult your doctor if your symptoms don't improve with changes in your eating habits or if you notice:
- Diarrhea
- Constipation
- Nausea or vomiting
- Weight loss
- Abdominal or rectal pain
- Persistent heartburn
- Blood in stools
- Fever

These symptoms may signal a more serious, underlying digestive condition.

Home remedies

To reduce excess gas

- Avoid foods that affect you the most. Common gas producers may include beans, lentils, peas, cabbage, onions, broccoli, cauliflower, bananas, raisins, prunes, whole-wheat bread, bran cereals or muffins, and carbonated drinks. This doesn't mean eliminating all of these foods from your diet, only the worst offenders.
- Temporarily cut back on high-fiber foods. Add them back gradually over weeks.
- Eat fewer fatty foods. They slow digestion, allowing food more time to ferment.
- Eat slowly. Eating when stressed or on the run can interfere with normal digestion.
- Take a short walk after meals. Exercise is good for your gut.
- Try low-lactose or lactose-free products (Lactaid, Dairy Ease) if dairy products are a problem.
- Try products containing simethicone (Gas-X, Mylanta Gas). They can break up the bubbles in gas.
- Try Beano. The natural enzyme in this product assists digestion by making certain foods more digestible and helping reduce intestinal gas.

To reduce belching

- Eat and drink slowly. Take your time and avoid gulping. Limit drinking through straws.
- Cut down on carbonated drinks and beer, which release carbon dioxide gas.
- Avoid chewing gum or sucking on hard candy.
- Don't smoke cigarettes, pipes or cigars.
- Manage stress, which may aggravate the nervous habit of swallowing air.
- Check your dentures. A poor fit may cause you to swallow excess air when eating.
- Avoid lying down immediately after you eat and take steps to treat your heartburn.

To reduce bloating

- Eat fewer fatty foods, which delay stomach emptying.
- Eat fewer gas-producing foods, including the ones listed previously. Also avoid chewing gum and hard candy.

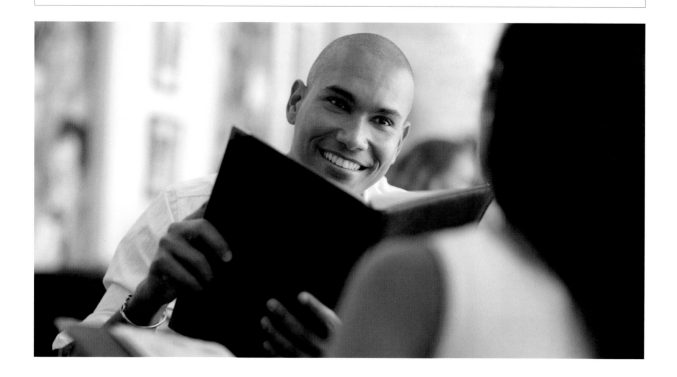

Gout

Gout is a complex form of arthritis characterized by sudden, severe attacks of pain, redness and tenderness in your body's joints. It may affect your feet, ankles, knees, hands and wrists, but most often occurs at the base of your big toe.

Gout develops when there is a high level of uric acid in your blood. As a result, sharp, needle-like urate crystals form in a joint or surrounding tissue that cause pain and swelling.

An acute attack of gout can wake you up in the middle of the night feeling like your big toe is on fire. The affected joint is hot, swollen and so tender that even the weight of the bedsheet on it seems intolerable.

Gout can affect anyone. In general, men are more likely to develop it. But women become increasingly susceptible to gout after they reach menopause.

Risk factors include obesity, excessive alcohol use, medical conditions such as high blood pressure, high cholesterol and diabetes, and having a family history of gout.

Medical help

Seek medical care immediately if you develop a fever and the joint becomes hot and inflamed. This can be a sign of infection.

Home remedies

Gout is treatable, and there are ways to reduce the risk that gout will recur. Here are guidelines that are recommended during a gout attack:

- Drink 8 to 16 cups of fluid each day, with at least half being water.
- Avoid alcohol.
- Limit your daily intake of protein from lean meat, fish and poultry to 4 to 6 ounces. Add protein to your diet with sources such as low-fat or fat-free dairy products and nut butters.
- Avoid foods that increase uric acid in your bloodstream. These include organ meats and certain seafoods (including anchovies, herring and sardines, mussels and scallops).
- Avoid products containing high-fructose corn syrup.
- Maintain a healthy weight.

Alternative treatments that may help

Since few alternative treatments have been studied in clinical trials, it's difficult to assess whether they're actually helpful for gout pain. The strategies that have been studied include:

- *Coffee.* Studies have found an association between coffee drinking — both regular and decaffeinated coffee — and lower uric acid levels in your blood, although no study has determined how or why coffee may have this effect.
- *Vitamin C.* Supplements containing vitamin C may reduce the levels of uric acid in your blood. However, vitamin C hasn't been studied specifically as a treatment for gout. Don't assume that if a little vitamin C is good for you, then lots is even better. In fact, megadoses of vitamin C may increase your body's uric acid levels. In place of supplements, you can increase your vitamin C intake by eating more fruits and vegetables, especially oranges.
- *Cherries.* Studies show an association between cherries and lower levels of uric acid in your blood, but it isn't clear if the cherries have any effect on the signs and symptoms. Eating cherries and other dark-colored fruits, such as blackberries, blueberries, raspberries and purple grapes, may be a safe way to supplement gout treatment, but discuss this strategy with your doctor first.

Headache

Headache is pain in any region of the head. It may be focused at one or both sides of the head, radiate across the head from a single point or have a viselike quality. The pain may be sharp, throbbing or dull. Symptoms may appear gradually or suddenly, and last for less than an hour or for several days.

Headaches are the most commonly reported medical complaint. They may point to an underlying medical condition but that situation is rare. About 90 percent of all headaches have no underlying cause. These so-called primary headaches may be the result of dysfunction or overactivity of the pain-sensitive features in your head — nerves, blood vessels, muscles — or of chemical activity in the brain.

The three best-known types of primary headache are:

Tension-type

This is the most common type of headache, and yet its causes aren't well-understood. The pain is generally mild to moderate and diffuse — many people describe feeling as if there's a tight band wrapped around their heads. Headaches can last from 30 minutes to a week.

Migraine

Migraines are chronic headaches that can last for hours or even days. The pain is moderate to severe, often with a pulsating or throbbing quality. Symptoms can be so severe that all you can think about is finding a dark, quiet place to lie down.

Some migraines are preceded, or accompanied, by sensory warning signs (auras), such as flashes of light, blind spots, or tingling in the arm or leg. The headache is often accompanied by nausea, vomiting and extreme sensitivity to light, odor and sound.

Cluster

A cluster headache is one of the most painful types of headache. Excruciating pain, generally located in or around the eye, strikes quickly, and usually without warning.

A striking feature of cluster headaches is that attacks occur in cyclical patterns, or clusters — giving the condition its name. Bouts (cluster periods) may last from weeks to months, followed by long periods of remission.

Medical help

If self-care doesn't help after one or two days, see your doctor. He or she will try to determine the type and cause of your headache and exclude other possible sources of pain with a variety of tests. Seek emergency care if the headache is the worst headache of your life or is associated with weakness, slurred speech or fainting.

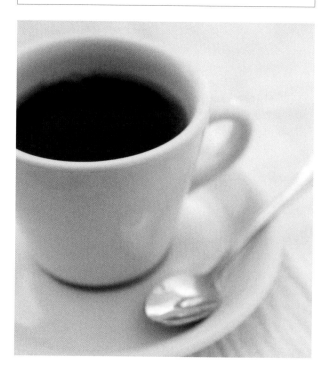

Home remedies

For tension-type headaches
- Try massage, hot or cold packs, a warm shower, rest, or other relaxation techniques.
- Try a low dose of aspirin (adults only), acetaminophen (Tylenol, others), ibuprofen (Advil, Motrin IB, others) or naproxen sodium (Aleve).
- Moderate exercise may help a tension-type headache.
- Poor posture may lead to tension headaches in some people. When sitting, don't slump your head forward. When standing, hold your shoulders back and your head high.
- Rub peppermint oil on your forehead and temples. Most peppermint oil contains menthol, which may ease pain.

For migraines
- Start treatment as soon as you feel a migraine coming — it's your best chance to stop the headache early. Use acetaminophen, ibuprofen or aspirin (adults only) at the recommended dosage.
- Some people can abort a migraine by going to sleep in a darkened room or by consuming caffeine (coffee or cola).
- Try muscle relaxation exercises, including meditation, yoga and progressive muscle relaxation. Or spend at least a half-hour each day doing something you find relaxing — listening to music, gardening or reading.

For cluster headaches
- Stick to a regular sleep schedule. Cluster periods may be triggered by changes in your normal sleep schedule.
- Avoid alcohol. Consuming alcohol usually triggers a headache when you're in a cluster period.
- Avoid being around volatile substances. Exposure to substances such as solvents, gasoline and oil-based paints may trigger headaches.
- Be cautious in high altitudes. The reduced oxygen levels may trigger headaches.
- Avoid tobacco. If you're prone to cluster headaches, it's best to stop smoking and avoid other tobacco products.
- Avoid nitrates. These compounds may trigger headaches for some people. Foods that contain nitrates include smoked and processed meats. Medications, such as nitroglycerin, also may contain nitrates.

Herbs, vitamins and minerals
- Evidence suggests that the herbs feverfew and butterbur may prevent or reduce the severity of headache symptoms. Don't take these if you're pregnant.
- A high dose of riboflavin (vitamin B-2) may help ease symptoms.
- Magnesium supplements seem to help some people with migraines, especially those with low levels of magnesium.
- Coenzyme Q10 is under study as a potential preventive agent for migraines. Research suggests it can decrease migraine frequency by about 30 percent.

Home remedies

Avoiding headache triggers

Some people can eliminate their headaches by avoiding headache triggers — certain foods, beverages, activities or environments that seem to produce a headache.

Headache triggers vary, but here are common examples:

- Red wine or other alcohol
- Caffeine
- Fermented, pickled or marinated food, aged cheese, bananas, citrus fruits, dried fruits, food additives and seasonings (sodium nitrite in hot dogs and luncheon meat, or monosodium glutamate in Chinese foods), nuts, peanut butter, and chocolate
- Smoking
- Stress or fatigue
- Depression or anxiety
- Lack of sleep
- Changing sleeping patterns or mealtimes
- Skipping meals
- Eyestrain
- Poor posture
- Weather, altitude or time zone changes
- Oral contraceptive use or hormone therapy
- Strong or flickering lights
- Strong odors, including perfumes, flowers or natural gas
- Polluted air or stuffy rooms
- Excessive noise

Caffeine and headaches

- A morning headache can occur, especially if you regularly consume four or more cups of caffeinated drinks each day. It may be a withdrawal headache, following a night without caffeine.
- Caffeine may also help. Some kinds of headaches cause blood vessels to widen. Caffeine temporarily causes them to narrow.
- So, for adults, if aspirin or acetaminophen (Tylenol, others) doesn't help, use a medicine that includes caffeine. But don't overdo it. Too much caffeine can cause jitteriness, rapid heart rate, sweating and, yes, withdrawal headaches.

Rebound headaches

Rebound headaches are caused by the frequent use of headache medication. Pain relievers can offer relief for occasional headaches, but if you take them more than a couple of days a week, you may trigger medication overuse (rebound) headaches.

How frequently rebound headaches occur depends on the type of overused drug. This happens because your body adapts to the medication.

- *Simple pain relievers.* Common drugs such as aspirin and acetaminophen (Tylenol, others) may contribute to rebound headaches — especially if you exceed the recommended daily dosages. Ibuprofen (Advil, Motrin IB, others) and naproxen sodium (Aleve) have a low risk of rebound headaches.
- *Combination pain relievers.* Over-the-counter drugs that combine caffeine, aspirin and acetaminophen (Excedrin, others) are common culprits of rebound headaches. Prescription medications such as Fioricet and Fiorinal also contain the sedative These medications put you at high risk of rebound headaches.
- *Migraine medications.* Migraine drugs linked to rebound headaches include triptans (Imitrex, Zomig, others) and certain ergots, such as ergotamine (Ergomar, others). They have a moderate risk of causing rebound headaches.
- *Opioids.* Painkillers derived from opium or from synthetic opium compounds, including combinations of codeine and acetaminophen (Tylenol with Codeine No. 3 and No. 4, others), have a high risk of rebound headaches.

To stop rebound headaches, reduce or stop taking pain medication. It's tough in the short term, but your doctor can help you beat rebound headaches for long-term relief.

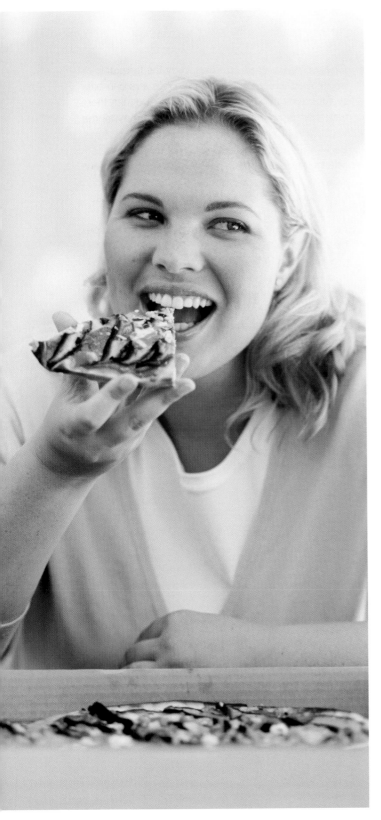

Heartburn

Heartburn is a burning sensation in your chest, just behind your breastbone. Often due to gastro-esophageal reflux disease (GERD), heartburn occurs when stomach contents back up into your esophagus. Sour taste and the sensation of food coming back into your mouth may accompany the sensation.

Heartburn often happens after you've eaten a meal, and it may occur at night. The pain usually worsens when you're lying down or bending over. It can be worsened or triggered by eating acidic or fatty foods.

Why does food back up into your esophagus? Normally, esophageal muscles contract in sequence, sending our food through the esophagus to the stomach. If the muscle is weak, stomach contents can wash back up (reflux), irritating the esophagus.

Occasional heartburn is common and no cause for alarm. Most people manage the discomfort on their own. More-frequent heartburn that interferes with your daily routine may be a symptom of something more serious that requires assistance from your doctor.

Medical help

Most problems with heartburn are occasional and mild. If you have severe or daily discomfort, don't ignore the symptoms. Left untreated, chronic heartburn can scar the lower esophagus and make swallowing difficult. In rare cases, severe heartburn leads to Barrett's esophagus, which may increase your risk of esophageal cancer.

Seek immediate medical attention if you experience chest pain, especially when accompanied by other signs and symptoms, such as shortness of breath or pain in the jaw or arm. These may be signs and symptoms of a heart attack.

Home remedies

Most people can manage the discomfort of heartburn with lifestyle changes and over-the-counter medications.

- *Maintain a healthy weight.* The pressure of excess pounds on your abdomen pushes up your stomach, causing acid to back up into your esophagus. If you are overweight or obese, work to slowly lose weight — no more than 1 or 2 pounds a week. Ask your doctor for help in devising a weight-loss strategy.
- *Avoid tightfitting clothing.* Clothes that fit tightly around your waist put pressure on your abdomen, helping force stomach acid to wash back into your esophagus.
- *Avoid foods and drinks that trigger heartburn.* Everyone has specific triggers. These may include fatty foods, alcohol, caffeinated or carbonated beverages, decaffeinated coffee, peppermint, spearmint, garlic, onion, cinnamon, chocolate, citrus fruits and juices, and tomato products.
- *Avoid big meals.* Avoid overeating by eating smaller, and more-frequent meals.
- *Delay lying down after a meal.* Wait at least two to three hours after eating before lying down to rest or take a nap.
- *Don't eat before bed.* Don't eat two to three hours before bedtime. Don't drink liquids or take pills 30 minutes to an hour before bedtime.

- *Elevate the head of your bed.* An elevation of about 6 to 9 inches at the head of your bed helps gravity work for you against stomach reflux. Place wood or cement blocks under the bedposts at the head of your bed. If it's not possible to elevate the bed frame, insert a wedge between the mattress and box spring that elevates your body from the waist up. Wedges are available at drugstores and medical supply stores.
- *Don't smoke.* Smoking interferes with proper function of the lower esophageal sphincter.
- *Use over-the-counter antacids occasionally.* These products can temporarily neutralize stomach acid and relieve mild heartburn. However, prolonged or excessive use of antacids containing magnesium can cause diarrhea. Calcium or aluminum-based products can lead to constipation.
- *Try other medications.* Products such as famotidine (Pepcid), omeprazole (Prilosec), cimetidine (Tagamet Hb) and ranitidine (Zantac) may relieve heartburn symptoms by reducing the production of stomach acid. These medicines are available in both over-the-counter and prescription strengths. Follow medication instructions about eating and drinking to maximize their effectiveness.

Heat exhaustion

Under normal conditions, the natural mechanisms that control your body temperature adjust well to the outside environment. Working hard in hot or humid conditions for prolonged periods, however, may overstress the systems, causing an excessive increase in body temperature.

Heat exhaustion may come on suddenly or may develop after days of heat exposure. Signs and symptoms include cool, moist skin with goosebumps when in the heat, heavy sweating, faintness, dizziness, fatigue, weak rapid pulse, muscle cramps, nausea, and headache.

What's heatstroke?

Heatstroke is a life-threatening condition that occurs when your body temperature reaches 104 F or higher. It's an escalation of two other heat-related health problems: heat cramps and heat exhaustion. With heatstroke, you stop sweating and your skin becomes hot, flushed and dry. You may feel confused and disoriented. Other signs and symptoms include rapid, shallow breathing, rapid heartbeat, headache, and muscle cramps or weakness.

Medical help

Untreated, heat exhaustion can progress to heatstroke. If you don't begin to feel better within 60 minutes, seek prompt medical attention. If you suspect heatstroke, call 9ll or emergency medical help immediately.

Home remedies

To avoid heat-related conditions:
- *Limit your exposure.* Avoid being outside during the hottest part of the day, which is generally from noon to 4 p.m. Reserve vigorous exercise or activity for early morning or evening. If possible, exercise in the shade.
- *Drink plenty of fluids.* Water and sports drinks are good options for staying hydrated. Avoid alcohol and caffeine, which can contribute to fluid loss.
- *Dress appropriately for the weather.* Wear loosefitting, lightweight, light-colored clothing.
- *Avoid hot and heavy meals.*
- *Pace yourself.* Let your body acclimate to the heat.
- *Find cover.* At the first sign of heat exhaustion, get out of the sun and rest in the shade or in an air-conditioned building.
- *Apply cool water to your skin.* If possible, take a cool shower or soak in a cool bath. Don't use alcohol on your skin.

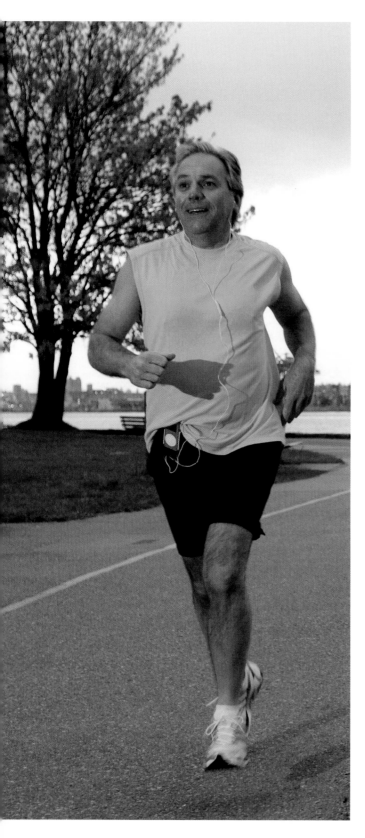

Heel pain

Your heels take a lot of punishment — every mile you walk puts heavy stress on each foot. Too much physical activity, poorly fitting shoes and excess weight can cause pain and inflammation.

Pain that develops directly under the heel is most often the result of plantar fasciitis. This is an inflammation of the plantar fascia, the fibrous tissue along the bottom of your foot that connects to your heel bone. Pain can also occur just behind the heel, where the Achilles tendon attaches to the heel bone (insertional Achilles tendinitis). Although the cause often isn't serious, heel pain can be severe and occasionally disabling.

Heel pain usually develops gradually, but can also occur suddenly and severely. Although both feet may be affected, it usually occurs in only one foot.

Pain tends to be worse when you get out of bed in the morning, and generally goes away as your foot limbers up. It can recur if you stand for a long time, get up from a sitting or lying position, climb stairs, or stand on tiptoes. A bone spur (usually painless) may form due to the tension on your heel bone.

Treatment generally involves relieving pain and inflammation. However, don't expect a quick cure. Relief may take six months or longer.

Medical help

If self-care measures aren't effective, or if you believe your condition may be caused by a foot abnormality, see your doctor.

Home remedies

To relieve heel pain:

- *Cut back on exercises such as jogging or walking, which impact the heel.* Substitute exercises that put less weight on your heel, such as swimming or bicycling.
- *Apply ice to the painful area.* Do this for up to 20 minutes after an activity to reduce inflammation.
- *Stretch your heel.* Stretching increases your flexibility. Stretching in the morning before you get out of bed helps reverse the tightening that occurs overnight. Stretch your heel after exercise, such as walking or running. See the stretches below.
- *Wear the right shoes.* Buy shoes with good heel and arch support and shock absorbency.
- *Experiment with inserts Try heel pads or cups that cushion and support your heel.*
- *Don't walk barefoot, especially on hard surfaces.* Going shoeless can aggravate heel pain.
- *Try nonprescription pain relievers.*
- *Lose weight.* If you're overweight, lose weight to reduce stress on your heel.

Heel exercises

These exercises stretch or strengthen your plantar fascia, Achilles tendon and calf muscles. The two exercises illustrated below are best done while seated.

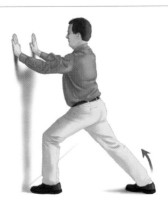

Calf stretch

1. Stand at arm's length from a wall or a sturdy piece of exercise equipment. Put your palms flat against the wall or hold on to the piece of equipment.
2. Keep one leg back with your knee straight and your heel flat on the floor.
3. Slowly bend your elbows and front knee and move your hips forward until you feel a stretch in your calf.
4. Hold this position for 30 to 60 seconds.
5. Switch leg positions and repeat with your other leg.

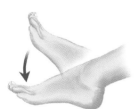

Active foot stretch

Stretch for 20 to 30 seconds up, then 20 to 30 seconds down, doing two or three repetitions. This exercise can be done multiple times a day before weight bearing.

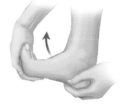

Passive foot stretch

Gently pull the top of your foot forward and hold stretch for 20 to 30 seconds, doing two or three repetitions. This exercise can be done two or three times each day.

Hemorrhoids

Hemorrhoids are dilated or enlarged veins in your anus. By age 50, about half of adults have experienced the itching, burning and discomfort that signals their presence. You may also notice small amounts of blood on toilet tissue or in the toilet bowl.

Hemorrhoids usually develop due to increased pressure, for example, as you strain to pass hard stools. Lifting heavy objects, obesity, pregnancy, childbirth, stress and diarrhea also can increase the pressure on these veins and lead to hemorrhoids.

There are two common types of hemorrhoids. An internal hemorrhoid develops within the anal canal. You can't see or feel it, and it usually doesn't cause any discomfort. An external hemorrhoid is under the skin around your anus. When irritated, it can itch and bleed.

In addition to hemorrhoids, bleeding from the rectum can occur for other reasons, some of which can be serious. Therefore, it's important not to dismiss all rectal bleeding as hemorrhoids.

Medical help

Hemorrhoids become most painful when a clot forms in the enlarged vein. If this happens, your doctor may prescribe a cream or suppository containing hydrocortisone to reduce the inflammation. Troublesome internal hemorrhoids may require surgery or other procedures to shrink or eliminate them.

Home remedies

Although uncomfortable, hemorrhoids are not a serious medical condition. You can temporarily relieve mild pain, swelling and inflammation with the following self-care measures:

- *Increase water and fiber.* Drink plenty of water each day and eat high-fiber foods such as wheat-bran cereal, whole-wheat bread, fresh fruits and vegetables.
- *Cleanse gently.* Bathe or shower daily to gently cleanse the skin around your anus. Regular soaking in a warm bath is best. Soap isn't necessary and may aggravate the irritation.
- *Stay active and exercise.* If you must sit or stand for long periods, try to take quick walks or frequent breaks.
- *Don't strain.* Try not to push during bowel movements or sit on the toilet for long periods of time.
- *Use moist wipes or wet toilet paper to wipe off stool.* Blot or pat dry.
- *Apply cold.* Use ice packs or cold compresses to relieve inflammation.
- *Try a product to soothe irritation.* To relieve mild itching and irritation, apply over-the-counter creams containing hydrocortisone or pads containing witch hazel or a topical numbing agent.
- *Taking fiber supplements (Citrucel, Metamucil).* These can help keep stools soft and regular.

Hiccups

Hiccups involve an involuntary contraction of your diaphragm — the thin muscular partition that separates your chest from your abdomen and plays an important role in breathing. Each involuntary contraction is followed by a sudden closure of your vocal cords, producing the characteristic "hic" sound.

A bout of hiccups usually lasts only a few minutes. Many people have home remedies for hiccups that they swear by. But in some people — about 1 in 100,000 — hiccups may persist for several months, no matter what remedies they may try to stop them.

Many factors may cause hiccups, but only rarely are hiccups a sign of an underlying medical condition.

Medical help

Make an appointment to see your doctor if your hiccups last more than 48 hours or if they are so severe that they cause problems with eating or breathing.

Home remedies

Although there's no surefire way to stop them, if you have a bout of hiccups that lasts longer than a few minutes, the following home remedies may provide relief:
- Swallow a teaspoon of sugar
- Breathe into a paper bag
- Gargle with ice water
- Hold your breath

Prevention
You may be able to decrease the frequency of hiccups by avoiding common hiccup triggers, such as:
- Large meals
- Carbonated beverages or alcohol
- Sudden changes in temperature
- Excitement or emotional stress

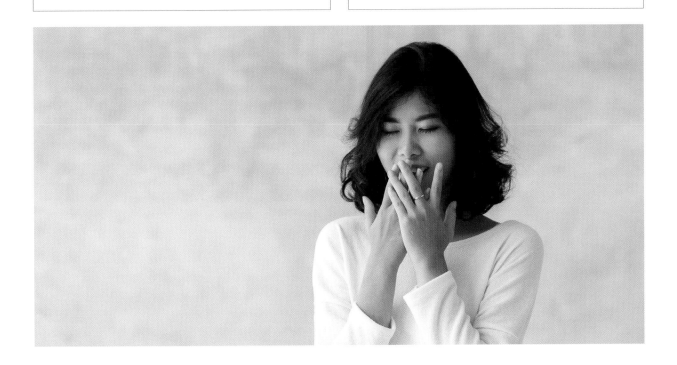

High blood pressure

Most people with high blood pressure (hypertension) don't experience any signs or symptoms, even if their blood pressure reaches dangerously high levels. That's why it's called a silent killer. Uncontrolled blood pressure can damage your arteries, heart, brain, kidneys and eyes. It increases your risk of serious health problems, including heart attack, stroke and kidney failure.

Blood pressure basics

Blood pressure is determined by the amount of blood your heart pumps and the amount of resistance to blood flow in your arteries. The more blood your heart pumps and the narrower your arteries, the higher your blood pressure.

Blood pressure is highest when your heart muscle contracts and pumps out blood — that's your systolic blood pressure. Between each contraction, your heart rests, lowering your blood pressure — that's your diastolic blood pressure. Your blood pressure readings have two numbers: the systolic pressure (top number) and diastolic pressure (bottom number).

Medical help

High blood pressure requires medical attention. See a doctor if you think you have high blood pressure. The doctor can determine if you need medication and, if so, which type may work best for you.

Know your numbers

Top number (systolic)	Bottom number (diastolic)	What it means	What to do
Below 120	and Below 80	Normal	Maintain or adopt a healthy lifestyle
120-139	or 80-89	Prehypertension	Adopt a healthy lifestyle*
140-159	or 90-99	Stage 1 hypertension	Lifestyle changes plus a medication†
160 or higher	or 100 or higher	Stage 2 hypertension	Lifestyle changes plus more than one medication

*These recommendations address high blood pressure as a single health condition. If you also have heart disease, diabetes, chronic kidney disease or certain other conditions, you'll need to treat your blood pressure more aggressively.

†If your blood pressure isn't normal, a healthy lifestyle — often times along with medication — can help bring it under control and reduce your risk of life-threatening complications.

Note: This chart applies to adults 18 and older. Numbers are in millimeters of mercury (mm Hg). Diagnosis is based on the average of two or more readings taken at two different visits, after the initial screening. If your readings fall into two different categories, your result is the higher category.

Based on American Heart Association, 2017

Home remedies

Lifestyle changes can help you prevent or control high blood pressure — even if you're taking blood pressure medication. Here's what you can do:

Eat healthy foods

Try the Dietary Approaches to Stop Hypertension (DASH) diet, which emphasizes fruits, vegetables, whole grains and low-fat dairy products. Get plenty of potassium, which can help control high blood pressure. Eat less saturated fat and total fat.

Limit salt

Salt causes the body to retain fluids and so, in many people, can raise blood pressure. Don't add salt to food. Avoid foods that include a lot of salt in processing, such as cured meats, snack foods, and many canned or frozen foods.

Maintain a healthy weight

If you're overweight, losing even 5 pounds may lower your blood pressure. In some people, weight loss alone is sufficient to avoid the need to take blood pressure medications.

Increase physical activity

Regular physical activity can help lower your blood pressure and keep your weight under control. Try to get at least 30 minutes of physical activity every day. Don't think you've got to run a marathon or join a gym. Consider moderate aerobic activity, such as walking or bicycling.

Don't smoke

Smoking tobacco products injures blood vessel walls and makes them less flexible (hardening of the arteries). If you smoke, ask your doctor to help you quit.

Limit alcohol

Even if you're healthy, alcohol can raise your blood pressure. If you choose to drink alcohol, do so in moderation — no more than one drink a day for women and anyone over age 65, and a limit of two drinks a day for men.

Manage stress

Reduce daily stress as much as possible. Get plenty of sleep. Practice healthy coping techniques, such as deep breathing.

Monitor your blood pressure

Home blood pressure monitoring can help you keep closer tabs on your blood pressure, indicate if your medication is working, and even alert you and your doctor to potential complications.

Eat dark chocolate

Certain compounds in dark chocolate can lower blood pressure slightly (milk chocolate does not have the same effect). Enjoy in moderation.

Try paced respiration

Paced respiration refers to slow, deep breathing. In various clinical trials, regular use of a nonprescription device (Resperate) that helps analyze and guide your breathing patterns was found to help lower blood pressure. However, some researchers have questioned whether this benefit is due to the device or simply a result of taking 15 minutes to relax.

High cholesterol

Cholesterol is a waxy substance that's found in the fats (lipids) in your blood and used by your body to build healthy cells. There are different types of cholesterol, including low-density lipoprotein (LDL, or "bad") cholesterol and high-density lipoprotein (HDL, or "good") cholesterol.

Problems occur when you regularly carry undesirable levels of cholesterol in your bloodstream: too much of one type, not enough of another type, or both. High levels of LDL cholesterol can cause fatty deposits to build up in your blood vessels. Eventually, these deposits restrict blood flow through your arteries. The lack of oxygen-rich blood to your heart increases the risk of heart attack. Decreased blood flow to your brain can cause a stroke.

What about triglycerides?

Triglycerides are a type of fat associated with blood cholesterol. When you eat, your body converts any calories it doesn't need into triglycerides. The triglycerides are stored in your fat cells, and later released as a source of energy between meals.

High triglyceride levels may be caused by excess weight and inactivity. People with high triglyceride levels often have high levels of LDL cholesterol as well. High triglyceride levels increase your risk of heart disease and stroke.

Medical help

Ask your doctor for a baseline cholesterol test at age 20 and then have your cholesterol retested at least every five years. If your test results aren't within desirable ranges, your doctor may recommend more-frequent measurements.

Know your numbers

Cholesterol and triglycerides are fats that circulate in your blood. In the past, the guidelines below were considered appropriate for most people:

Type of blood fat	Typical goals
Total cholesterol	Below 200
LDL ("bad") cholesterol	Below 100 (below 70 if you're at very high risk of a heart attack)
HDL ("good") cholesterol	Men: 40 or higher Women: 50 or higher
Triglycerides	Below 150

Numbers are in milligrams per deciliter of blood (mg/dL).

However, one size doesn't fit all. Your goals may differ, especially if you have risk factors for heart disease and other conditions. The American Heart Association recommends to get your cholesterol checked and to talk to your doctor about your numbers and how they impact your specific overall risk.

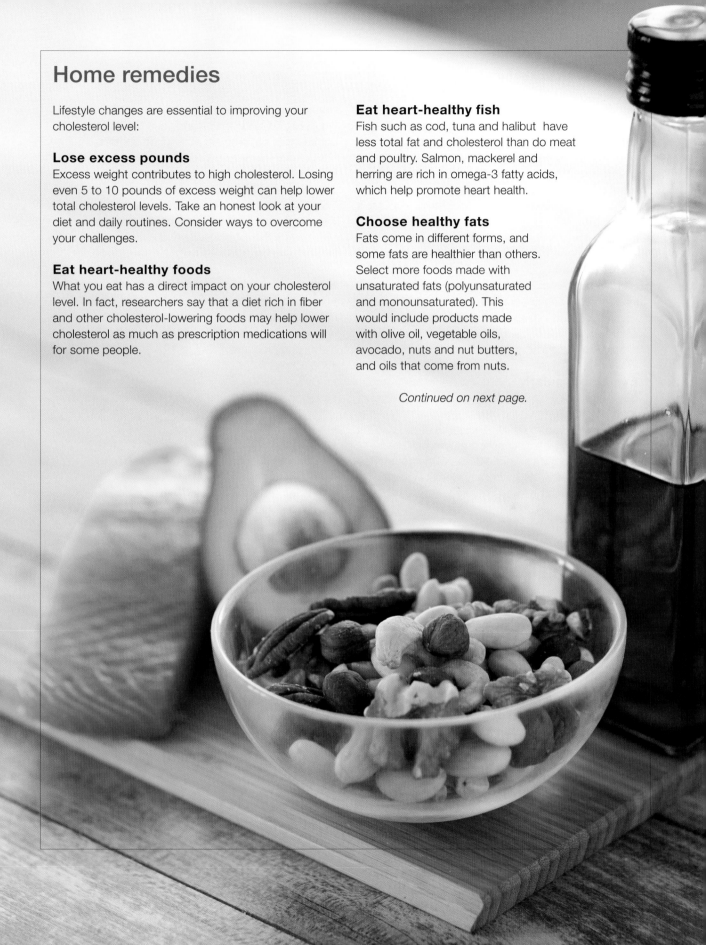

Home remedies

Lifestyle changes are essential to improving your cholesterol level:

Lose excess pounds

Excess weight contributes to high cholesterol. Losing even 5 to 10 pounds of excess weight can help lower total cholesterol levels. Take an honest look at your diet and daily routines. Consider ways to overcome your challenges.

Eat heart-healthy foods

What you eat has a direct impact on your cholesterol level. In fact, researchers say that a diet rich in fiber and other cholesterol-lowering foods may help lower cholesterol as much as prescription medications will for some people.

Eat heart-healthy fish

Fish such as cod, tuna and halibut have less total fat and cholesterol than do meat and poultry. Salmon, mackerel and herring are rich in omega-3 fatty acids, which help promote heart health.

Choose healthy fats

Fats come in different forms, and some fats are healthier than others. Select more foods made with unsaturated fats (polyunsaturated and monounsaturated). This would include products made with olive oil, vegetable oils, avocado, nuts and nut butters, and oils that come from nuts.

Continued on next page.

Eat fruits and vegetables

Fruits and vegetables are the foundation of a healthy diet, as well as for successful weight loss. Explore different types and varieties for appealing tastes and textures.

Drink alcohol in moderation

In some studies, moderate use of alcohol has been linked with higher levels of HDL cholesterol — but this benefit isn't strong enough to recommend alcohol for anyone who doesn't drink already.

Don't smoke

Stopping smoking can improve your HDL cholesterol level. And the benefits don't end there. Within one year, your risk of getting heart disease is half that of a smoker's. Within 15 years, your risk is similar to that of someone who's never smoked at all.

Exercise regularly

Regular exercise can help improve cholesterol levels. Try to include 30 to 60 minutes of exercise daily. Take a brisk walk. Ride your bike. Swim laps. If you can't fit a single session into your schedule, you can get similar benefits from several 10-minute workouts. See your doctor before beginning any type of vigorous exercise program.

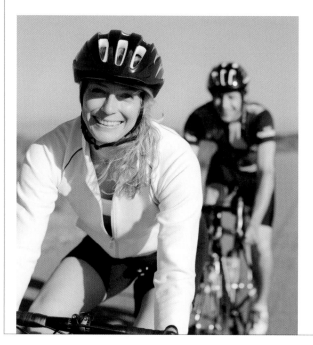

Select whole grains

Whole grains are packed with essential vitamins, minerals and fiber that promote heart health. Choose whole-grain breads, pasta and flour. Brown rice, oatmeal and oat bran are other good choices.

Eliminate trans fats

Trans fats are often found in margarines and commercially baked cookies, crackers and snack cakes. Trans fats are double trouble for heart health, raising LDL ("bad") cholesterol levels and lowering HDL ("good") cholesterol levels.

Experiment with natural products

Although few natural products have been proven to reduce cholesterol, some may be helpful. You might consider trying these cholesterol-lowering supplements and products:

- Artichoke
- Barley
- Blond psyllium (found in seed husk and products such as Metamucil)
- Flaxseed
- Garlic
- Oat bran (found in noninstant oatmeal and whole oats)
- Plant sterols and stanols. These compounds include beta-sitosterol (found in oral supplements and some margarines, such as Promise Activ) and sitostanol (found in oral supplements and some margarines, such as Benecol). They help block the absorption of cholesterol and can lower LDL ("bad") cholesterol.

A caution on red yeast rice

You may have heard of a supplement for reducing cholesterol called red yeast rice. The Food and Drug Administration has warned that some brands of red yeast rice contain a naturally occurring form of lovastatin, a prescription drug used to lower cholesterol. This can be unsafe, since there's no way to determine the quantity or quality of the lovastatin in the red yeast supplements.

Hives

Hives are raised, red, often itchy welts of various sizes that appear and disappear on your skin. They tend to occur in batches and last anywhere from a few minutes to several days. Hives are more common on areas of the body where clothes rub the skin.

Angioedema, a similar kind of swelling, causes large welts just below your skin, especially near your eyes and lips, but also on your hands and feet and inside your throat.

Hives and angioedema are a result of your body releasing a natural chemical called histamine in your skin. Allergies to foods, drugs, insect bites, infections, illness, pollen, cold and heat, and emotional distress may trigger this reaction. However, for many people the cause of hives remains unclear.

In most cases, hives and angioedema are harmless and leave no lasting marks. However, serious angioedema may cause swelling in your throat or tongue that blocks your airway, causes loss of consciousness and can be life-threatening.

Medical help

Seek emergency care if you feel lightheaded or have difficulty breathing or if hives continue to appear for more than a couple of days. Also seek medical attention if the hives are associated with other signs and symptoms, such as fever or joint pains.

Home remedies

If you're experiencing mild hives or angioedema, these tips may help relieve your symptoms:

- *Look for triggers.* Try to identify and avoid substances that irritate your skin or that cause an allergic reaction. These may include foods, medications, pollen, pet dander, latex and insect stings.
- *Use an over-the-counter antihistamine.* A non-prescription oral antihistamine, such as cetirizine (Zyrtec), diphenhydramine (Benadryl) or loratadine (Claritin) may help relieve itching.
- *Apply cool, wet compresses.* Covering the affected area with bandages and dressings can help soothe the skin and prevent scratching.
- *Take a comfortably cool bath.* To relieve itching, sprinkle the bath water with baking soda, uncooked oatmeal or colloidal oatmeal — a finely ground oatmeal made for bathing (Aveeno).
- *Wear loose, smooth-textured cotton clothing.* Avoid clothing that's rough, tight, scratchy or made from wool, to reduce irritation.
- *Keep a diary.* If you suspect foods are causing the problem, keep a food diary. Be aware that food labels may list some ingredients under less common names.
- *Reduce stress.* Practicing stress management techniques may help avoid a reaction.

Hoarse voice

You've likely had days when your voice sounds excessively husky, raspy or weak. You may have even lost your voice for a short time (laryngitis). This occurs when your vocal cords become swollen or inflamed and are no longer able to vibrate normally. They produce unnatural sounds, or possibly no sound at all.

In addition to difficulty speaking, you may feel some pain or have a raw, scratchy throat. Your voice may change pitch, sounding higher or lower than normal.

A common cause of hoarseness is infection, especially a viral infection of the upper respiratory system, such as a cold or flu. You can also become hoarse from vocal strain caused by yelling or overusing your voice. Other causes include allergies, smoking, and the chronic reflux of stomach acid into your esophagus.

Hoarseness and laryngitis may be short-lived (acute) or long lasting (chronic). Most acute cases are not serious, but persistent hoarseness may signal a serious underlying condition.

Medical help

If hoarseness lasts for more than four weeks, seek medical help. Seek immediate medical attention if your child makes noisy, high-pitched breathing sounds when inhaling, drools more than usual, has trouble swallowing and has a body temperature higher than 103 F. These signs and symptoms may indicate epiglottitis, which requires medical attention.

Home remedies

The following steps may reduce strain on your voice and relieve the symptoms of hoarseness and laryngitis:

- *Rest your voice.* Limit how much talking you do. Whispering puts even more strain on your vocal cords than does normal speech.
- *Drink lots of warm, noncaffeinated fluids.* Fluids help keep your throat moist. Also try sucking on lozenges, gargling with salt water or chewing a piece of gum.
- *Inhale steam.* Breathe in steam from a bowl filled with hot water. (Never inhale steam directly from water as it boils.) Lean over the container with a towel draped over your head to help catch the steam. Breathing deeply during a hot shower also may help.
- *Use a humidifier to moisturize the air.* Follow the manufacturer's instructions to clean the humidifier and prevent bacterial buildup.
- *Avoid clearing your throat.* This action irritates your vocal cords.
- *Stop drinking alcohol and smoking, and avoid exposure to smoke.* Alcohol and smoke dry your throat and irritates your vocal cords.
- *Avoid decongestants.* These medications can dry out the throat.

Impetigo

Impetigo is a highly contagious skin infection that usually appears on the face. The infection begins when common bacteria penetrate your skin through a cut, scratch or insect bite. Although a much less common occurrence, impetigo may also develop in healthy skin.

The infection appears as red sores that blister briefly, ooze for several days and then form a sticky, yellowish-brown crust. Scratching or touching the sores can spread the infection on your body or to other people.

Other signs and symptoms of impetigo include:
- Itching
- Painless, fluid-filled blisters
- In a more serious form, painful fluid- or pus-filled sores that turn into deep ulcers

Impetigo is more common among young children. In adults, it develops mostly as a complication of other skin problems, such as dermatitis or breaks in the skin. There's a small chance of kidney damage or rheumatic fever resulting from the infection.

Home remedies

Good hygiene is essential for preventing impetigo and limiting its spread. For minor infections that haven't spread to other parts of your body, try the following:

- *Soak the affected areas of skin with a vinegar solution.* Combine 1 tablespoon of white vinegar with 1 pint of water. Soak the areas for 20 minutes. This makes it easier to gently remove the scabs.
- *After washing the area, apply over-the-counter antibiotic ointment 3 or 4 times daily.* Wash the skin before each application, and pat it dry. Keep the sores and skin around them clean.
- *Avoid scratching or touching the sores as much as possible until they heal.* Apply a nonstick dressing to the infected area to help keep impetigo from spreading. Children's fingernails should be trimmed to help reduce damage from scratching.
- *Don't share towels, clothing or razors with others.* Change your bathroom linens daily.

Medical help

See your doctor if the infection doesn't appear to be improving. Antibiotics are often prescribed that may speed healing of the sores and limit the spread of infection.

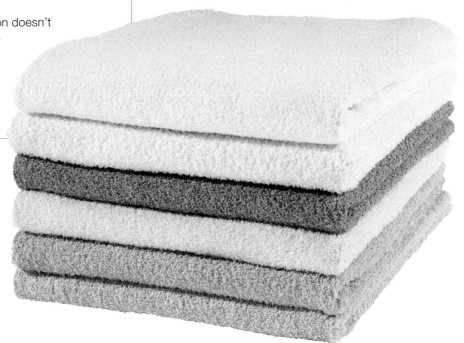

Incontinence

Urinary incontinence means a loss of bladder control, resulting in accidental and untimely leakage. It's a common problem that may be caused by everyday behaviors, underlying medical conditions or physical problems.

Your concerns may range from occasional minor leaks or dribbles to sudden, strong urges to urinate. Types of incontinence include:

- **Stress incontinence.** This is a loss of urine when you exert pressure on your bladder from coughing, sneezing, laughing, exercising or lifting.
- **Urge incontinence.** This is a sudden, strong urge to urinate, often with only seconds or minutes to reach a toilet.
- **Overflow incontinence.** An inability to empty your bladder results in frequent and constant dribbling of urine.
- **Functional incontinence.** Some people have a physical or mental impairment, for example, arthritis or dementia, that prevents them from getting to the toilet on time.

Other causes of incontinence include over-hydration or dehydration, drinking alcohol or caffeine, taking certain medications, and consuming substances that irritate the bladder.

Medical help

You may feel uncomfortable discussing incontinence. But if incontinence is frequent or is affecting your quality of life, don't hesitate to discuss your concerns with your doctor.

Home remedies

Lifestyle changes work well for treating certain types of urinary incontinence:

Bladder training

This involves learning to delay urination every time you get the urge to go. You may start by trying to hold off for 10 minutes. The goal is to lengthen the time between toilet trips until you're urinating every two to four hours. Bladder training may also involve double voiding — urinating, then waiting a few minutes and trying again to empty your bladder more completely.

Scheduled toilet trips

The idea here is timed urination — going to the toilet according to the clock rather than waiting for the need to go. Try to go every two to four hours.

Fluid and diet management

You may be able to simply modify your daily dietary habits to regain control of your bladder. You may need to cut back on or avoid alcohol, caffeine or acidic foods.

Pelvic floor muscle exercises

These exercises, called Kegels, strengthen the abdominal muscles that help control urination. Imagine that you're trying to stop the flow of urine. If you're using the right muscles, you'll feel a pulling sensation. Pull in your pelvic muscles and hold for a count of three. Relax for a count of three. Work up to 10 to 15 repetitions each time you exercise. Do Kegel exercises at least three times a day. It may take up to 12 weeks before you notice an improvement in bladder control.

Indigestion

Indigestion, also called upset stomach or dyspepsia, is a general term that describes discomfort in your upper abdomen. Indigestion isn't a disease but rather a collection of signs and symptoms, such as bloating, belching, nausea and feeling uncomfortably full after eating a meal.

There are many possible causes of indigestion. Some are related to your lifestyle and others to what you eat and drink. Anxiety, smoking, high stress, mealtime habits (such as eating too quickly) and digestive conditions, such as ulcers or gallstones, also may cause indigestion.

Sometimes people with indigestion also experience heartburn, but heartburn and indigestion are two separate conditions. Heartburn is a pain or burning feeling in the center of your chest (see pages 93-94).

Although the condition is common, how you experience indigestion may differ from how others do. Fortunately, you may be able to prevent or treat symptoms with self-care.

Medical help

Mild indigestion is usually nothing to worry about. Consult your doctor if discomfort persists for more than two weeks. Contact your doctor right away if indigestion is severe or accompanied by:
- Weight loss or loss of appetite
- Vomiting
- Black, tarry stools
- Yellow coloring in the skin and eyes (jaundice)

Home remedies

Dietary changes and healthy lifestyle choices may help prevent mild indigestion.
- *Eat smaller, more-frequent meals.* Choose mostly fresh vegetables, fruits and whole grains. Chew your food slowly and thoroughly.
- *Avoid triggers.* Common triggers of indigestion include fatty and spicy foods, carbonated beverages, caffeine, alcohol, and smoking.
- *Maintain a healthy weight.* Extra pounds put pressure on your abdomen and may cause stomach acid to back up into your esophagus.
- *Exercise regularly.* Exercise helps you keep off extra weight and promotes better digestion. With your doctor's OK, aim for 30 to 60 minutes of physical activity on most days of the week.
- *Manage stress.* Get plenty of sleep. Spend time doing things you enjoy. Practice relaxation techniques such as meditation or yoga.
- *Reconsider your medications.* With your doctor's approval, stop or cut back on aspirin or other anti-inflammatory drugs that can irritate your stomach lining. If that's not an option, be sure to take these medications with food.
- *Drink herbal tea with peppermint.* Some people find relief from indigestion with peppermint, although more research is needed to determine its effectiveness.

Ingrown hairs

An ingrown hair occurs when the tip of a hair curls back and grows into the skin, causing inflammation and irritation. This is more likely to happen after hair has been cut close to the skin, for example, by shaving or tweezing. The sharp tip of hair that's formed by these actions can penetrate the skin more easily than can uncut hair.

Ingrown hairs most commonly appear in the beard area of males, including the chin, cheeks and, especially, the neck. In females, the most common areas are the armpits, pubic area and legs. Signs and symptoms may include:

- Localized pain
- Areas of small, dry, rounded bumps
- Small, pus-filled, blister-like lesions
- Skin darkening
- Itching

Ingrown hairs are most likely to occur in black males, ages 14 to 25. But an ingrown hair candevelop in anyone who shaves, tweezes, waxes or uses electrolysis to remove hair.

Medical help

See your doctor if ingrown hairs are a chronic problem for you.

Home remedies

Follow these steps to release ingrown hairs.
- Wash the affected area using a washcloth or soft-bristled toothbrush — using a circular motion — for several minutes before shaving and at bedtime
- Use a sterile needle, inserting it under hair loops, to gently lift hair tips that are embedded in your skin

Prevention

Of course, not removing hair is one way to avoid an ingrown hair. If that's not an option, there are hair-removal methods that make ingrown hairs less likely. If you shave:
- Wet the hair or whiskers to be removed with warm water
- Avoid close shaves
- Use a lubricating shave gel
- Use a single-blade razor
- Use a sharp blade
- Don't pull your skin taut while shaving
- Shave in the direction of hair growth
- Rinse the blade after each stroke
- Apply cool compresses to the shaved area when you're finished

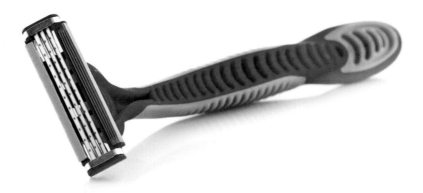

Ingrown toenails

An ingrown toenail is a common condition in which the corner or side of one of your toenails grows into the soft flesh of the toe. The result is pain, redness, swelling around a nail and, sometimes, an infection. An ingrown toenail usually develops on your big toe.

Common causes include wearing shoes that crowd your toenails, cutting your toenails too short or not straight across, injuring your toenail, or having unusually curved toenails.

Usually, an ingrown toenail is taken care of before any serious problems can develop. But, if left untreated, tissue surrounding the toe and the underlying bone can become infected.

Medical help

If the pain of an ingrown toenail is severe or spreading, your doctor can take steps to relieve discomfort and help you avoid complications. Also seek medical attention if you experience areas of pus or redness on the toe that appears to be spreading or if you have diabetes or poor blood circulation.

Home remedies

You can treat most ingrown toenails at home. Here's how:

- *Soak your feet in warm salt water.* For every pint of water, add 1 teaspoon of salt. Soak your feet for 15 to 20 minutes three times a day. Soaking reduces swelling and relieves tenderness.
- *Place cotton under your toenail.* Put fresh bits of cotton or dental floss under the ingrown edge after each soaking. This will help the nail eventually grow above the skin edge. Change the cotton or floss daily until the pain and redness subside.
- *Use a topical antibiotic.* Apply an antibiotic ointment and bandage to the tender area.
- *Choose sensible footwear.* Consider wearing open-toed shoes or sandals until your toe feels better.
- *Check your feet.* If you have diabetes, check your feet daily for signs of ingrown toenails or other foot problems.
- *Take pain relievers.* If the pain is severe, take over-the-counter pain relievers, such as ibuprofen (Advil, Motrin IB, others), naproxen sodium (Aleve) and acetaminophen (Tylenol, others), to relieve the pain until you can make an appointment with your doctor.

Insect bites and stings

Signs and symptoms of an insect bite are caused by the injection of venom or other substances into your skin. The venom sometimes triggers an allergic reaction. The severity of your reaction depends on how sensitive you are to the venom and whether you've been bitten or stung more than once.

Most reactions are mild, causing a slight itching or stinging sensation and mild swelling that disappear within a day or so. A delayed reaction, which can happen hours or even days later, may cause fever, hives, painful joints and swollen glands.

Only a small percentage of people develop severe reactions to insect venom. For information on severe allergic reactions, see page 186. Signs and symptoms may include:
- Nausea
- Facial swelling
- Difficulty breathing
- Abdominal pain
- Deterioration of blood pressure and circulation

Bites from bees, hornets, wasps, yellow jackets and fire ants are typically the most troublesome. Bites from mosquitoes, ticks, biting flies and some spiders also can cause reactions, but these are generally milder.

Mosquito bites

There's no denying that mosquito bites are annoying. You're most likely to be bitten at dawn or dusk, when the insects are most active. You can take steps to keep mosquitoes at bay, but no method is foolproof. Telltale signs and symptoms — redness, swelling and itching — may not appear for up to two days after the bite.

Mosquito bites may sometimes transmit serious diseases, such as Zika virus, West Nile virus, chikungunya virus, malaria and dengue fever. Signs and symptoms of more serious infection include fever, severe headache, body aches, lethargy, confusion and sensitivity to light. Such signs and symptoms require prompt medical attention.

Spider bites

Most spider bites produce harmless itching or stinging that goes away in a day or two. Only a few spiders are dangerous to humans, including the black widow — known for the red hourglass marking on its belly — and the brown recluse — with its violin-shaped marking on its top.

These two spiders prefer warm climates and dark, dry places, such as closets, woodpiles and outdoor toilets. Signs of a black widow bite start with slight swelling and redness at the bite. Within hours, however, you may experience intense pain, stiffness, chills, fever, nausea and severe abdominal pain.

If bitten by either of these spiders, seek emergency care immediately.

Tick bites

Some ticks carry infections and their bites can transmit bacteria that cause illness. For information on tick bites, see page 173.

Medical help

If you have any breathing problems; swelling of the lips, tongue or throat; faintness; confusion; rapid heartbeat; or hives after a sting, seek emergency care. Less severe allergic reactions include nausea, intestinal cramps, diarrhea or swelling larger than 2 inches wide at the site. See your doctor promptly if you have any of these symptoms.

Home remedies

Most insect bites and stings feel unpleasant but are generally harmless and easily treated at home. The following steps may help relieve discomfort.

- In the case of a sting, brush off the stinger from the skin with a straight-edged object. Don't pull out the stinger. This may release more venom.
- Wash the bite or sting area with soap and water.
- Apply a cold pack or cloth filled with ice to reduce the pain and swelling.
- Apply 0.5 or 1 percent hydrocortisone cream, calamine lotion, aloe vera, or a paste of baking soda and water to the bite or sting several times daily until your symptoms go away. To make a baking soda paste, mix 1 teaspoon water with 3 teaspoons baking soda.
- Take an antihistamine (Benadryl, Chlor-Trimeton, others) to reduce itching.

Mosquito bites

The preceding steps can help relieve itching. To reduce your risk of getting bit by mosquitoes:

- Avoid unnecessary outdoor activity when mosquitoes are most active, at dawn, dusk and early evening.
- Wear light-colored, long-sleeved shirts and long pants outdoors.
- Use mosquito repellent that contains DEET. Don't apply DEET on the hands of young children and don't use DEET on infants under 2 months of age.
- Apply permethrin-containing mosquito repellent to your clothing or buy clothing with permethrin in it.

Spider bites

If bitten by a black widow or brown recluse spider:

- Use soap and water to clean the wound and skin around the spider bite.
- Slow the venom's spread. If the spider bite is on an arm or leg, tie a snug bandage above the bite and elevate the limb to help slow or halt the venom's spread. Ensure that the bandage is not so tight that it cuts off circulation in your arm or leg.
- Use a cold cloth at the spider bite location. Apply a cloth dampened with cold water or filled with ice.
- Seek immediate medical attention. Treatment may require antivenom medication.

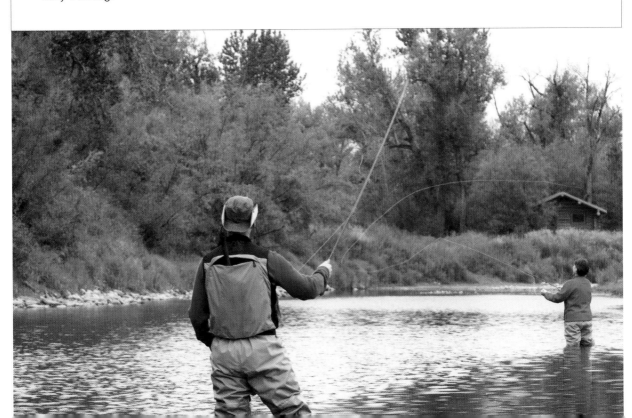

Although antihistamine-based medications may improve mild symptoms of insomnia, they aren't likely to help for longer than a couple of weeks. Some common nonprescription sleep aids include:

- *Diphenhydramine (Sominex, others).* These products may cause dry mouth, dizziness, prolonged drowsiness and memory problems. They're not recommended if you're pregnant or breast-feeding or you have a history of glaucoma, heart problems or an enlarged prostate.
- *Doxylamine (Unisom).* This medication may cause periods of prolonged drowsiness. It may not be safe if you're pregnant or breast-feeding, or if you have a history of asthma, bronchitis, glaucoma, peptic ulcers or an enlarged prostate gland. While taking this type of medication, don't drive or attempt other activities that require alertness.

What about antihistamines?

Antihistamines may help you fall asleep for a few nights — but routine use of antihistamines for insomnia isn't recommended.

Antihistamines induce drowsiness by counteracting histamine, a chemical produced by the central nervous system. In fact, most nonprescription sleep aids contain antihistamines. These products are intended to be used for only two to three nights at a time, such as when stress, travel or other disruptions prevent you from falling asleep. You can quickly develop a tolerance to the sedative effects of antihistamines — so the longer you take them, the less likely they are to make you sleepy.

Medical help

If, after a week or two, you still have trouble sleeping, see your doctor. Doctors generally don't recommend taking sleeping pills for more than a few days. However, they may recommend sleeping pills as temporary help until other treatments begin to work. If your doctor thinks you may have a sleep disorder other than insomnia, you may be referred to a sleep center for special testing.

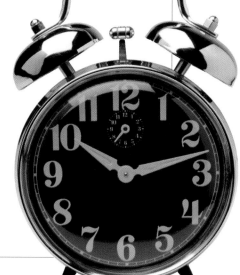

Irritable bowel syndrome

Irritable bowel syndrome (IBS) is a common disorder of the gastrointestinal tract. IBS can be stressful, painful, disruptive and at times embarrassing. But it does not indicate cancer, and it's not life-threatening.

It's not known what causes IBS, but the condition affects muscle contractions in the intestines and colon. If you have IBS, the contractions can feel stronger, last longer and are often relieved — at least temporarily — by passing stool.

You're more likely to have IBS if you are young, are female and have a family history of IBS. Researchers are studying whether this family history relates to a genetic inheritance, to a shared environment or to a combination of both.

Irritable bowel syndrome doesn't cause inflammation or tissue changes, nor does it increase your risk of colorectal cancer. Many people discover that signs and symptoms improve as they learn to control the condition through the proper management of diet, lifestyle and stress.

Signs and symptoms

Signs and symptoms of IBS vary widely, and can resemble those of many other diseases. Abdominal pain or discomfort, diarrhea or constipation, bloating, abdominal gas, and mucus in the stool are all signs of IBS.

Like many people, you may experience only mild signs and symptoms, but for some, these problems are disabling. IBS tends to be a chronic condition, with periods of more-severe symptoms alternating with periods of low-level symptoms or no symptoms.

Triggers

For reasons that aren't clear, if you have IBS you may be reacting strongly to certain stimuli that may have little effect on other people. Common triggers for IBS may include:

- **Foods.** Symptoms may worsen when you eat certain foods, including chocolate, milk and alcohol. Be aware that if you experience cramping and bloating after eating dairy products, food with caffeine or sugar-free candy, the problem may be an intolerance to sugar (lactose), caffeine or the artificial sweeteners sorbitol and mannitol.
- **Stress.** Many people with IBS find their symptoms worsen or become more frequent during stressful events, such as changes in the daily routine or during family arguments. However, while stress may aggravate the symptoms, it doesn't cause them.
- **Hormones.** Although it's not understand why, IBS is more than twice as common in women than in men. Women may find their symptoms are worse during or around their menstrual periods, and sometimes symptoms improve with menopause.
- **Other illnesses.** Infection, such as an acute episode of infectious diarrhea, can sometimes trigger IBS symptoms. The symptoms may last for years but eventually improve.

Medical help

Because symptoms of IBS may mimic those of more-serious medical problems, such as cancer, gallbladder disease and ulcers, see your doctor if self-care measures don't help within a couple of weeks. You may need testing if the following occurs: new onset after age 50, weight loss, rectal bleeding, fever, nausea or recurrent vomiting, abdominal pain (especially if it's not completely relieved by bowel movement), or persistent diarrhea.

Home remedies

Simple lifestyle changes may provide some relief from irritable bowel syndrome (IBS):

- *Experiment with fiber.* Fiber can be a mixed blessing. Although it helps reduce constipation, it can also make gas and cramping worse. The best approach is to gradually increase the fiber in your diet over a period of weeks. Examples of foods that contain fiber are whole grains, fruits, vegetables and beans. Some people do better taking a fiber supplement, such as Metamucil or Citrucel, which causes less gas and bloating. Be sure to introduce a supplement gradually and drink plenty of water every day.

- *Avoid problem foods.* If certain foods make your signs and symptoms worse, don't eat them. Common culprits include alcohol, chocolate, caffeinated beverages, carbonated drinks, and sugary drinks and sweeteners. High-fructose foods or sweeteners such as sorbitol or mannitol can aggravate symptoms. If gas is a problem, foods that may trigger symptoms include beans, cauliflower, cabbage and broccoli. Fatty foods also may be a problem.

- *Take care with dairy products.* If you're lactose intolerant, try using an enzyme product that breaks down lactose, or substituting yogurt for other dairy products as a source of calcium. Consuming milk products in small amounts or combining them with other foods also may help. Some people may need to eliminate dairy completely.

- *Eat at regular times.* Not skipping meals and eating at about the same time each day helps you stay regular. If you have diarrhea, eating small, frequent meals may help ease bouts. If you're constipated, eating high-fiber foods may help move food through your intestines.

- *Drink plenty of liquids.* Water is best. Caffeinated or carbonated drinks may make symptoms worse.

- *Exercise regularly.* Exercise stimulates normal intestinal contractions and helps relieve stress. If you've been inactive, start slowly and gradually and work up to 30 minutes a day most days of the week. If you have medical concerns, check with your doctor before starting an exercise program.

- *Try peppermint.* In some studies, symptoms of IBS improved significantly among people taking peppermint capsules. In other studies, there was no benefit. Peppermint contains menthol, which is thought to relax stomach muscles and speed passage of food through the stomach.

- *Eat yogurt and other probiotics.* Probiotics are foods containing "good" bacteria similar to those normally found in your body. These bacteria help maintain a microorganic balance in your intestinal tract. Probiotics include yogurt, miso, tempeh, and some juices and soy drinks. They're available in supplement form.

Jammed finger

A jammed finger is typically a sprain to the joint (knuckle) of the finger. There may also be a small fracture or dislocation of the joint. The injury can be extremely painful, and the joint usually becomes swollen.

A jammed finger is a common sports injury. For example, your fingertip receives the full impact of a hard-hit baseball, basketball rebound or volleyball spike. A jammed finger may also result for other reasons. You reach out your arm to break a fall, and your finger jabs into the ground. The result is often a jammed finger.

This type of injury usually heals quickly if there is no fracture, although the pain may linger for months when direct pressure is applied to the finger.

Home remedies

To treat a jammed finger:
- Ice the finger with a cold pack for 15 minutes. Placing your finger in ice water works, too.
- Elevate your hand to reduce swelling.

To protect the finger during use:
- "Buddy tape" the injured finger to an adjacent finger. Use a self-adhesive wrap to tape above and below the finger joint — for example, tape the index finger to middle finger or ring finger to small finger.

Medical help

Seek medical care if:
- Your finger appears deformed
- You cannot straighten your finger
- The area becomes hot and inflamed and you develop a fever
- Swelling and pain become significant or persistent
- The finger becomes numb, and turns white or pale

Children require medical care because damage to the growth plate of a finger bone can lead to long-term deformity.

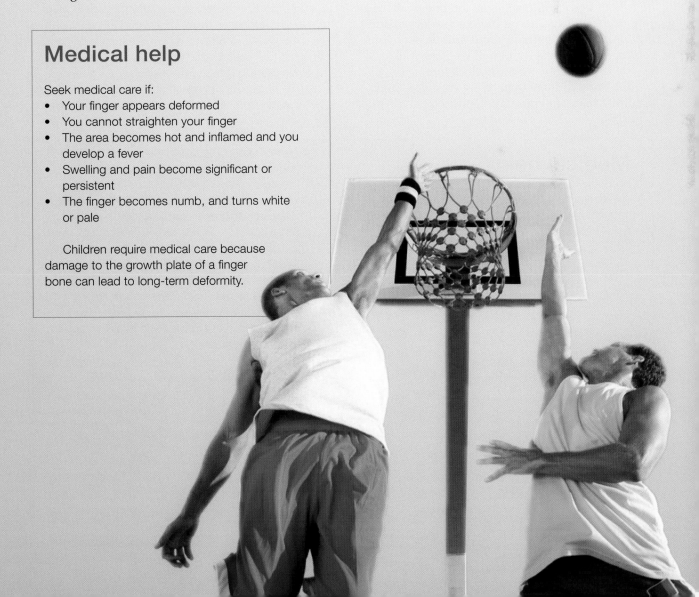

Jet lag

If you've traveled by air to another location in a different time zone, you're probably familiar with that dragged-out feeling called jet lag. The sleep disorder is caused by a disruption of your body's internal clock or circadian rhythm — which signals when it's time to be awake and when it's time to sleep. The more time zones you cross, the more likely you are to have jet lag.

Symptoms of jet lag may vary but can include:

- Disturbed sleep
- Daytime fatigue
- Difficulty concentrating
- Stomach problems
- Not feeling well
- Muscle soreness

Your body will readjust at the rate of about an hour a day. Thus, if you change four time zones, your body may require about four days to get back into its usual rhythm. Flying eastward — and resetting your body clock forward — is often more difficult than flying westward and adding hours to your day.

Medical help

Jet lag is a temporary condition. But if you are a frequent traveler and struggle with jet lag, you may benefit from seeing a sleep specialist.

Home remedies

To reduce or prevent jet lag:

- *Reset your body's clock.* Several days in advance of your departure, adopt a waking-sleeping cycle that's closer to what you'll have at your destination.
- *Drink plenty of fluids and eat lightly.* Drink extra liquids during your flight to avoid dehydration, but limit beverages with alcohol and caffeine. They increase dehydration and may disrupt your sleep.
- *Avoid taking a sleeping pill on the flight over.* However, taking an over-the-counter sleep aid for the first three nights after reaching your destination may help you to adjust.
- *Switch immediately to local time.* On arrival at your destination, reset your watch to local time. If possible, don't plan a hectic schedule on the first day. Consider arriving at your destination in the evening, if traveling eastward.
- *Be outside.* Try to spend some time outside in the day time. Exposure to natural light can help with resetting your body's clock and adjusting to jet lag.
- *Try melatonin.* The use of melatonin has its pros and cons. The latest research suggests that melatonin does indeed aid sleep during times when you wouldn't normally be resting, making it of particular benefit for people with jet lag. Small doses — as little as 0.5 milligram — seem just as effective as larger doses. Take melatonin 30 minutes before you plan to sleep or ask your doctor about the proper timing. Avoid alcohol when taking melatonin. Side effects are uncommon but may include dizziness, head-ache and loss of appetite, and possibly nausea and disorientation.

Kidney stones

Kidney stones are small, hard deposits that form inside your kidneys. The stones are made of mineral and acid salts. Kidney stones have many causes. For example, they can form when your urine becomes concentrated, allowing minerals to crystallize and stick together.

Passing a stone through the urinary tract can be painful. The pain typically starts in your side or back, just below your ribs, and moves to your lower abdomen and groin. The location of pain may change as the stone moves through your tract.

Factors that increase your risk of kidney stones include:

- Family or personal history of kidney stones
- Being adult
- Being male
- Dehydration
- Eating a high-protein, high-sodium and high-sugar diet
- Obesity
- Digestive diseases and surgery that can cause changes in the digestive process
- Other medical conditions, including gout, hyperparathyroidism and certain urinary tract infections

Medical help

Make an appointment with your doctor if you have any signs or symptoms that worry you. Seek immediate medical attention if you experience:

- Pain so severe that you can't sit still or find a comfortable position
- Pain accompanied by nausea and vomiting
- Pain accompanied by fever and chills
- Blood in your urine

Home remedies

One of the most effective ways to reduce your risk of kidney stones is to drink more fluids — ideally water — to increase your urine output to about 2.5 liters in a 24-hour period. Aim to drink enough fluid that your urine is nearly clear or has only a light yellow tinge. Here are other measures that may help prevent kidney stones:

- *Avoid foods and beverages that contain high-fructose corn syrup.*
- *Limit sodium.* Reduce your daily salt intake.
- *Avoid calcium-containing antacids.*
- *Watch your meat consumption.* Limit intake of beef, pork and poultry to no more than 4 to 6 ounces a day.
- *Eat moderate amounts of dairy products.* This means keeping between one and three servings each day.
- *Eat fewer oxalate-rich foods.* If you tend to form calcium oxalate stones, your doctor may recommend restricting foods rich in oxalates. These include rhubarb, beets, okra, spinach, Swiss chard, sweet potatoes, tea, chocolate and soy products.
- *Drink tea.* Drinking a cup of black tea or green tea each day could reduce your risk of kidney stones. One study found that a group of women who drank the most black tea had a slightly lower risk of kidney stones. Although this study was not a rigorous one, if you currently enjoy tea, there's a chance that continuing to drink it may help reduce your risk of kidney stones.
- *Drink lemon juice and orange juice.* The citric acid levels in lemon juice and orange juice may reduce calcium levels in your urine, leading to fewer kidney stones, even though no studies have proved this theory. If you enjoy drinking water flavored with lemon or drinking orange juice every morning, you may actually be helping to reduce your risk.

Knee pain

Knees are a common location of pain. The pain may be related to an injury, overuse or changes that occur in your body at different stages of life. The locations and severity of knee pain may vary depending on the cause of the problem.

Injuries

Knee injuries are often complex. A knee bears a lot of weight and isn't designed to handle sideways stress. The injury may affect any of the muscles, tendons or fluid-filled sacs (bursae) that surround your knee as well as the bones, cartilage and ligaments that form the joint itself. The signs and symptoms vary widely. Pain may be the result of:
- Trauma or a blow to the knee
- Sudden turning, pivoting, stopping and cutting from side to side
- Awkward landings from a fall or from jumping

While self-care measures may be helpful for minor injuries, more-serious injuries such as ruptured ligaments or tendons may require surgical repair.

Knee overuse

Any repeated stress or overuse of your knees can result in pain. Knee overuse conditions are often sports-related. Pain from overuse is common in adolescents with rapidly growing bones. Overuse pain also occurs more readily in older adults, typically because of degeneration in the knee joint.

Pain from knee overuse is generally more minor than is pain from an inury, and it usually responds well to the self-care measures below.

Medical help

Seek medical care immediately if:
- The injury produces intense pain and a large amount of swelling, and the knee doesn't function properly or feel stable
- The pain follows a popping sound or a snapping or locking feeling
- You're suddenly unable to straighten your knee (locking)

Home remedies

The key to treating knee pain is to break the cycle of inflammation that begins right after the injury, decreasing the swelling and pain. Simple self-care measures can be remarkably effective in ending this cycle:
- *Follow the instructions for P.R.I.C.E.* See page 157.
- *Take an anti-inflammatory medication.* Nonsteroidal anti-inflammatory medications such as ibuprofen (Advil, Motrin IB, others) and naproxen (Aleve) help relieve inflammation. However, seek medical advice if you have any kidney problems or stomach problems before using NSAIDs.
- *Flex and straighten your leg gently every day.* If it's difficult to move your knee, have someone help you at first. Try to straighten it and keep it straight.
- *Avoid strenuous activity until your knee heals.* Start nonimpact exercises slowly.
- *Avoid squatting, kneeling, or walking up and down hills.* Stress of this kind may aggravate your knee injury.

Prevention
Regular exercise strengthens your knee muscles and helps prevent knee pain. Bend your knee only to a 90-degree angle during exercise. Don't do deep squats or deep lunges.

Lactose intolerance

Lactose intolerance means that you aren't able to fully digest lactose, a natural sugar in milk and other dairy products. It's a problem that becomes increasingly common with age. The condition usually is not dangerous, but its symptoms can be uncomfortable.

The problem behind lactose intolerance is your body's deficiency of lactase — an enzyme that breaks down lactose during the digestive process. In fact, many people have low levels of lactase, but only a segment of this larger group have associated signs and symptoms. These are the individuals who have, by definition, lactose intolerance.

Signs and symptoms of lactose intolerance usually begin 30 minutes to two hours after eating or drinking foods that contain lactose. Common signs and symptoms include:

- Diarrhea
- Nausea
- Abdominal cramps
- Bloating and gas

Symptoms of lactose intolerance are usually mild, but they may sometimes be severe. It may not be necessary to completely avoid all dairy foods. Most people with lactose intolerance can enjoy some milk products without symptoms — they just choose what to eat with caution.

Medical help

There's currently no way to boost your body's production of the lactase enzyme. However, make an appointment with your doctor if you or your child has any signs or symptoms that worry you.

Home remedies

People with lactose intolerance can reduce their signs and symptoms by carefully selecting and limiting dairy products. Simple ways to adjust your diet include:

- *Choosing smaller servings of dairy.* Sip small servings of milk — up to 4 ounces at a time. The smaller the serving, the less likely it is to cause gastrointestinal problems.
- *Experimenting with an assortment of dairy products.* Not all dairy products have the same amount of lactose. For example, hard cheeses, such as Swiss or cheddar, have small amounts of lactose and generally cause no symptoms. You may be able to tolerate products such as yogurt, because bacteria used in the culturing process naturally produce the enzyme lactase.
- *Buying products that contain lactase, such as Lactaid and Dairy-Aid.* You can find these products at most supermarkets in the refrigerated dairy section.
- *Using lactase enzyme products.* Over-the-counter tablets or drops containing the lactase enzyme may help you digest dairy products.

A caution on dairy-free diets

It's OK to experiment with a dairy-free diet, but you run the risk of a calcium deficiency, especially if started at an early age. This is important because too little calcium can lead to weakened bones over time.

To combat this, talk with your doctor about how to get adequate calcium, through alternative sources of dietary calcium, through supplements, or both.

Leg swelling

Swelling can occur in any part of your legs, including feet, ankles, calves or thighs. The swelling may result from fluid buildup or from inflammation in injured or diseased tissues or joints.

Many causes of leg swelling are relatively harmless in the long term, but sometimes, the swelling may be a sign of a more serious disorder, such as heart disease or a blood clot.

Some generalizations that may help you determine the cause of leg swelling include:

- Swelling in only one leg is more likely related to a condition in that leg alone.
- Swelling in both legs is more likely caused by a condition not directly related to the legs, such as prolonged standing or sitting.
- Leg swelling usually isn't the only sign of a serious disorder. For example, leg swelling related to heart disease is likely to occur along with shortness of breath or chest pain.
- Leg swelling from a blood clot usually appears suddenly and for no obvious reason. The clots often cause an aching pain deep in the calf or inner thigh. The leg may also be cool and pale.

Medical help

Swelling in your legs can be a sign of a more serious condition. Seek medical care immediately if you have unexplained, painful swelling in your legs or if a swollen leg becomes warm, red and inflamed. Also see your doctor if the swelling remains despite self-care.

Home remedies

To help prevent or remedy occasional leg swelling:

- Lose weight and limit your salt intake.
- Elevate your legs to a level above your heart for 15 to 20 minutes every few hours to let gravity help move fluid toward your heart.
- During periods of prolonged sitting and travel, try to walk around frequently and stretch your legs.
- Consider using compression stockings, especially when you're on your feet for long periods of time or while traveling on an airplane. A compression level of 10 to 20 millimeters of mercury (mm Hg) or higher is recommended.

Lice

Lice are tiny parasitic insects that feed on your blood. They are easily spread through personal contact and by sharing belongings such as combs, clothing and bedding.

Several types of lice exist, named for the areas of the body where they prefer to feed: head lice, body lice and pubic lice, commonly called crabs. Lice live only one to two days off the body.

Signs and symptoms include intense itching, tickling sensations and small, red bumps on the scalp, neck and shoulders. The eggs, resembling tiny pussy willow buds, can be found on hair shafts. Eggs (nits) hatch in eight to nine days. With body lice, some people develop hives while others have abrasions from scratching.

Head lice are easiest to see at the nape of the neck and over the ears. Body lice are difficult to find because they burrow into the skin, but may be detected in the seams of underwear.

Scabies

Other unwelcome visitors may be tiny burrowing mites that cause an itchy condition called scabies, marked by thin, irregular burrow tracks on your skin made up of tiny blisters or bumps. Scabies is highly contagious and can spread quickly through physical contact. Medicated cream applied to your skin can kill the mites, although you may experience some itching for several more weeks.

Medical help

Consult your doctor before using products on a child younger than 2 months or if you're pregnant. The Food and Drug Administration (FDA) cautions that products containing lindane can cause serious side effects, even when used as directed.

Home remedies

These steps may help you eliminate lice infestations:

- *Use lotions and shampoos.* Several over-the-counter lotions and shampoos (Nix, Rid, others) are designed to kill lice. Apply the product according to package instructions, and don't rewash hair for one to two days after treatment. You may need to repeat the treatment in seven to 10 days. These lotions and shampoos typically aren't recommended for children under age 2. It's best to treat everyone in the household who's infested at the same time, as well as preventively treat those who are in close contact.
- *After shampoo treatment, rinse your hair with vinegar.* Grasp a lock of hair with a cloth saturated with vinegar and strip the lock downward to remove nits. Repeat until you've treated all the hair in this way. Or soak hair with vinegar and leave it on for a few minutes before combing. Then towel-dry the hair.
- *Comb wet hair.* Use a fine-toothed or nit comb to physically remove the lice from wet hair. Repeat every three to four days for at least two weeks. This method may be used in combination with other treatments and is usually recommended as the first line of treatment for children under age 2.
- *Wash contaminated items.* Wash bedding, stuffed animals, clothing and hats with hot, soapy water — at least 130 F — and dry them at high heat for at least 20 minutes.
- *Seal unwashable items.* Place in an airtight bag for two weeks.
- *Vacuum.* Give the floor and upholstered furniture a good vacuuming.
- *Wash combs and brushes.* Use hot, soapy water — at least 130 F — or soak combs and brushes in rubbing alcohol for an hour.

Menopause

Menopause is the permanent end of menstruation and fertility, defined as occurring 12 months after your last menstrual period. Some women reach menopause in their 30s or 40s, while others do so in their 50s or 60s. The average age for women in the United States is 51.

Menopause is a natural biological process, not a medical illness. Even so, the physical and emotional symptoms of menopause may disrupt your sleep, sap your energy, and trigger feelings of sadness and loss.

Hormonal changes cause the physical symptoms, but mistaken beliefs are partly to blame for many emotional ones. First, menopause doesn't mean the end is near — you've still got as much as half your life to go.

Second, menopause will not snuff out your femininity and sexuality. In fact, you may be one of many women who find it liberating to enjoy intimacy without having to worry about pregnancy and periods.

Most important, even though menopause is not an illness, you shouldn't hesitate to get treatment for severe symptoms.

Signs and symptoms often appear long before you "hit" menopause. They include:
- Irregular periods
- Decreased fertility
- Vaginal dryness
- Hot flashes
- Sleep disturbances
- Mood swings
- Increased abdominal fat
- Thinning hair
- Loss of breast fullness

Medical help

Vaginal bleeding after menopause is not normal and should be promptly evaluated by your doctor. The cause of bleeding may be entirely harmless, but postmenopausal bleeding has a number of serious causes, including cancer.

Stages of menopause

Because the transition occurs over months and years, menopause is commonly divided into these stages:
- **Perimenopause.** You begin to experience menopausal signs and symptoms, even though you still menstruate. Your hormone levels rise and fall unevenly, and you may have hot flashes and other symptoms. This may last four to eight years or longer. During this time, it's still possible to get pregnant, but not likely.
- **Postmenopause.** Once 12 months have passed since your last period, you've reached menopause. In the postmenopausal years that follow, your ovaries produce less of the sex hormones and don't release eggs.

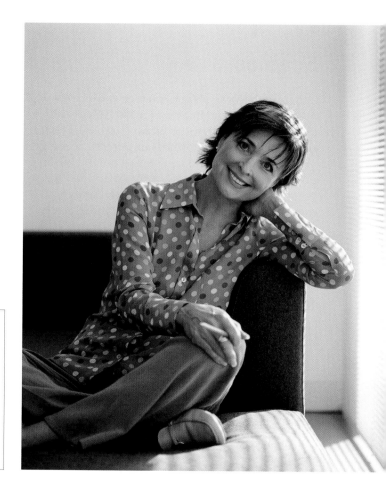

Home remedies

Fortunately, many signs and symptoms of menopause are temporary. The following steps may help reduce or prevent their effects.

Eat well

Eat a balanced diet that includes a variety of fruits, vegetables and whole grains and that limits saturated fats, oils and sugars. Include 1,200 to 1,500 milligrams of calcium and 800 international units of vitamin D a day.

Optimize your sleep

If you have trouble sleeping, avoid caffeinated beverages and don't exercise right before bedtime.

Exercise regularly

Get at least 30 minutes of moderately intense physical activity on most days to help protect against many conditions associated with aging. More-vigorous exercise for longer periods may provide further benefit and is particularly important if you're trying to lose weight and reduce stress.

Decrease vaginal discomfort

For vaginal dryness or discomfort with intercourse, use over-the-counter water-based vaginal lubricants (Astroglide, K-Y Jelly), moisturizers (Replens, Vagisil) or vaginal estrogen. Staying sexually active also helps.

Cool hot flashes

To cope with hot flashes, get regular exercise, dress in layers and try to pinpoint what triggers your hot flashes. Triggers may include hot beverages, spicy foods, alcohol, hot weather and even a warm room. Other remedies you might try include:

- *Black cohosh.* Studies show mixed results for black cohosh reducing menopausal symptoms, such as hot flashes. When taken short term, it appears to have a low risk of side effects. Don't take it for more than six months.
- *Isoflavones.* Soy is a common source of isoflavones, compounds with weak estrogen-like effects. These compounds may help with hot flashes. Study results regarding their safety and effectiveness are mixed. If you've had breast cancer, talk to your doctor before taking soy supplements.
- *Flaxseed.* Flaxseed is a source of phytoestrogens as well as omega-3 fatty acids. Some research suggests daily consumption of flaxseed improves mild menopause symptoms, such as hot flashes. Flaxseed is a healthy alternative to other fats and it's safe. However, it shouldn't be taken in large amounts by people who take warfarin (Coumadin).

Practice relaxation techniques

Techniques such as deep breathing, guided imagery, yoga and meditation don't directly target the hormonal fluctuations of menopause, but they may help you cope with mood swings, stress and sleep disturbances.

Menstrual cramps

If you're a woman, chances are you have dealt with menstrual cramps — even if you've never heard of the medical term for them: *dysmenorrhea.* Dull, throbbing or cramping pains develop in your lower abdomen and may extend to the lower back and thighs. Some women also have nausea, vomiting, diarrhea, sweating or dizziness.

Many women experience painful cramps just before or during their menstrual period. The discomfort may be merely annoying. But for some women, the pain they live with for a few days every month is severe enough to affect their mood and disrupt activities.

Many experts believe that cramping is a result of severe contractions of the uterus, which constrict blood vessels feeding the uterus. Menstrual cramps may also be caused by gynecologic conditions such as endometriosis and uterine fibroids.

Menstrual cramps tend to lessen with age and often disappear following childbirth.

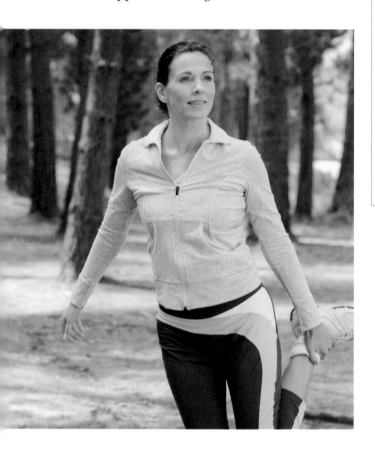

Medical help

Talk to your doctor if the cramping pain is severe or associated with a fever, or if the pain lasts several days a month and disrupts your life. Also see your doctor if you have nausea and vomiting or unusual vaginal discharge or odor.

Home remedies

To relieve or prevent menstrual cramps, try the following:

- *Pain relievers.* Nonsteroidal anti-inflammatory drugs, such as aspirin, ibuprofen (Advil, Motrin IB, others), naproxen (Aleve) and acetaminophen (Tylenol, others), taken as directed from the start of cramps until the cramps go away will relieve pain in most women. Girls under age 18 should not use aspirin.
- *Heat.* Try soaking in a warm tub or applying a heating pad on your lower abdomen.
- *Exercise.* Many women find that exercise helps lessen the symptoms of menstrual cramps.
- *Dietary supplements.* Some studies have indicated that vitamin E, thiamin, omega-3 and magnesium supplements may help reduce the symptoms of menstrual cramps.

Morning sickness

Morning sickness refers to nausea that occurs during pregnancy. The name is a misnomer, however, because morning sickness can strike at any time of the day (or even at night).

Morning sickness affects an estimated 50 to 90 percent of pregnant women. It's most common during the first trimester, but for some women morning sickness lingers throughout the pregnancy.

The condition is distressful and uncomfortable but is generally harmless. Medical treatment isn't usually necessary, although various home remedies often help relieve the nausea.

Medical help

Contact your doctor if, during periods of morning sickness:
- Nausea or vomiting is severe
- You pass only a small amount of urine or it's dark in color
- You can't keep down liquids
- You feel dizzy or faint when you stand up
- Your heart races
- You vomit blood

Home remedies

To help relieve morning sickness:
- *Choose foods carefully.* Opt for foods that are high in carbohydrates, low in fat and easy to digest. Salty foods are sometimes helpful, as are foods that contain ginger — such as ginger lollipops. Avoid greasy, spicy and fatty foods.
- *Snack often.* Before getting out of bed in the morning, eat a few soda crackers or a piece of dry toast. Nibble throughout the day, rather than eating three large meals. An empty stomach may aggravate nausea.
- *Drink plenty of fluids.* Sip water or ginger ale. It may also help to suck on hard candy, ice chips or ice pops.
- *Pay attention to situations that trigger nausea.* Avoid foods or smells or environments that seem to make your nausea worse.
- *Get plenty of fresh air.* Weather permitting, open the windows in your home or workplace. Take a daily walk outdoors.
- *Take care with prenatal vitamins.* If you feel queasy after taking prenatal vitamins, take the vitamins at night or with a snack. It may also help to chew gum or suck on hard candy after taking your vitamin. If these steps don't help, ask your doctor about switching to a type of prenatal vitamin that doesn't contain iron.
- *Try ginger.* A few studies suggest that ginger may help ease nausea from pregnancy. Ginger supplements are generally considered safe when taken in small amounts for a short time. However, it takes a few days for the ginger to work. Before taking the supplement, it may be best to talk with your doctor.

Motion sickness

Any type of transportation can cause motion sickness — boat, plane, train or automobile. Symptoms may strike suddenly, building from a feeling of unease to a cold sweat, dizziness and then vomiting.

Typically, you start feeling better as soon as the motion stops. The more you travel, the more easily you'll adjust to the motion.

You may be able to escape motion sickness by planning ahead. When you travel, reserve seats where motion is felt least:

- **By ship.** Request a cabin in the front or middle of the ship, or on the upper deck.
- **By plane.** Ask for a seat over the front edge of a wing. Once aboard, direct the air vent flow to your face.
- **By train.** Take a seat near the front and next to a window. Face forward.
- **By automobile.** Drive or sit in the front passenger's seat.

Medical help

If you're prone to severe motion sickness, talk with your doctor about prescription medications such as scopolamine (Transderm Scōp) before traveling. The drug offers 72-hour protection from motion sickness, although it can cause dry mouth and other side effects.

Home remedies

If you're susceptible to motion sickness:

- Focus on the horizon or on a distant, stationary object. Don't read.
- Keep your head still, while resting against a seat back.
- Don't smoke or sit near smokers.
- Breathe plenty of fresh air.
- Avoid spicy or greasy foods and alcohol. Don't overeat.
- Take an over-the-counter motion sickness drug such as meclizine (Bonine) or dimenhydrinate (Dramamine, Dramamine Less Drowsy Formula) before your outing.
- Consider scopolamine (Transderm Scōp), available in a prescription adhesive patch. Several hours before you plan to travel, apply the patch behind your ear for 72-hour protection. Talk to your doctor before using the medication if you have health problems such as asthma, glaucoma or urine retention.
- Eat dry crackers or drink a carbonated beverage to help settle your stomach if you become ill.

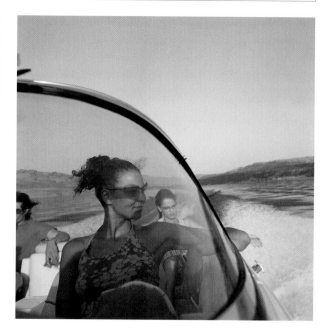

Muscle strain

A muscle can become strained or pulled — or even torn — when it is stretched unusually far or abruptly. This type of injury may also happen when muscles suddenly and powerfully contract.

Muscle strains often occur in the lower back, in the hamstring muscle in the back of your thigh, or in the shoulder. A slip on the ice or lifting from an awkward position may cause the muscle strain. Strains can vary in their severity:

- **Mild.** Causes pain and stiffness when you move. Symptoms will last a few days.
- **Moderate.** Causes small muscle tears and more-extensive pain, swelling and bruising. Pain may last one to three weeks.
- **Severe.** Muscle is torn or ruptured completely. You may have significant internal bleeding, swelling and bruising around the muscle. The muscle may not function at all. Seek immediate medical attention.

Home remedies

To relieve symptoms of muscle strain:
- Follow the instructions for P.R.I.C.E. (see page 157). The earlier the treatment, the speedier and more complete your recovery.
- For extensive swelling, use cold packs several times each day throughout your recovery.
- Don't apply heat when the area is still swollen.
- Avoid the activity that caused the strain while the muscle heals.
- Use over-the-counter pain medications as needed, such as ibuprofen (Advil, Motrin IB, others), naproxen (Aleve) and acetaminophen (Tylenol, others). Avoid using aspirin in the first few hours after the strain because aspirin may make bleeding more extensive. Don't give aspirin to children.

Medical help

Seek medical help immediately if the area quickly becomes swollen and is intensely painful. Call your doctor if the pain, swelling and stiffness don't improve in two to three days or if you suspect a ruptured muscle or broken bone.

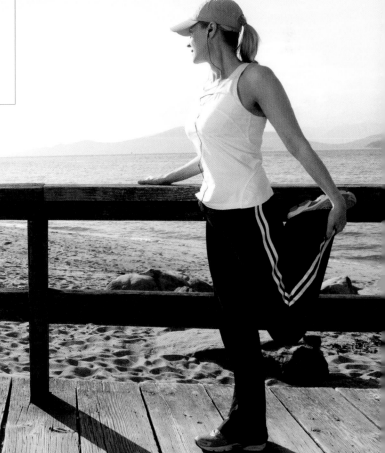

Nausea and vomiting

Nausea is a queasy feeling in your stomach that can be caused by many things, including a viral infection, headache, gallstones, food poisoning, motion sickness, radiation therapy, general anesthesia, pregnancy, dizziness, fear and anxiety, overeating, and exposure to strong odors. The list of potential causes goes on and on.

Nausea often, but not always, leads to vomiting — a violent, forceful ejection of stomach contents through your mouth. With repeated vomiting, there comes a risk of dehydration and losing important electrolytes.

Nausea and vomiting are common and uncomfortable but generally not serious. Infectious causes, such as viruses, can cause nausea and can also be associated with vomiting. Diarrhea, abdominal cramps, bloating and fever may accompany this condition.

Medical help

Contact your doctor if you're unable to drink anything for 24 hours, if vomiting persists beyond two or three days, if you become dehydrated, or if you vomit blood. Signs of dehydration include excessive thirst, dry mouth, little or no urination, severe weakness, dizziness, or lightheadedness. Vomiting may be a warning of more-serious underlying problems such as a concussion, gallbladder disease, ulcers, bowel obstruction or meningitis.

Home remedies

If a viral infection is the culprit, nausea and vomiting may last from a few hours to two or three days. Diarrhea and mild abdominal cramping also are common. To stay comfortable and prevent dehydration while you recover, try the following:

- Don't eat or drink anything for a few hours until your stomach has had time to settle.
- Try ice chips or small sips of weak tea, broths, clear soda (such as 7Up or Sprite) or noncaffeinated clear sports drinks to prevent dehydration. Consume 2 to 4 quarts (eight to 16 glasses) of liquid for 24 hours, taking frequent, small sips.
- Try adding semisolid and low-fiber foods gradually — but stop eating if the vomiting returns. Try soda crackers, gelatin, plain toast, eggs, rice or chicken.
- Avoid dairy products, caffeine, alcohol, nicotine, and fatty or highly seasoned foods for a few days.

Infant care
Most babies spit up food at least occasionally. Vomiting is a more forceful and disturbing action to your baby. It may lead to dehydration and weight loss if it's persistent.

- To prevent dehydration, let the baby's stomach rest for 30 to 60 minutes and then offer small amounts of liquid. If you're breast-feeding, let your baby nurse smaller amounts more frequently. Offer bottle-fed babies a small amount of formula or an oral electrolyte solution such as Pedialyte.
- If the vomiting doesn't recur, continue to offer small sips of liquid or the breast every 15 to 30 minutes.

Neck pain

Neck pain may involve muscles and nerves as well as cervical vertebrae and the disks that cushion them. Fortunately, most causes of neck pain aren't serious and can be treated with self-care.

Common causes of neck pain include:

- **Poor posture.** Whether leaning over a computer or hunched over a workbench, poor posture can strain muscles.
- **Muscle strain.** Overuse, such as twisting and turning your head, can trigger muscle strains. Even gritting your teeth can strain neck muscles.
- **Worn joints.** Your neck joints tend to experience wear and tear with age, which can cause osteoarthritis.
- **Nerve compression.** A so-called "pinched nerve" can occur when the space around your neck's vertebrae is reduced.
- **Injury.** Whiplash injuries, when the head is jerked sharply back and forth, stretches the soft tissues of the neck beyond their typical range of motion.
- **Disease.** Neck pain may be a symptom of disease, such as rheumatoid arthritis or meningitis.

Medical help

Sometimes neck pain can signify something more serious. Seek immediate medical care if you experience:

- Shooting pain into your shoulder or down your arm
- Numbness or loss of strength in your arms or hands
- Change in bladder or bowel habits
- Inability to touch your chin to your chest

Home remedies

Self-care measures to relieve neck pain include:

- *Pain relievers.* Try over-the-counter pain relievers, such as aspirin, ibuprofen (Advil, Motrin, others), naproxen (Aleve) and acetaminophen (Tylenol, others).
- *Alternate heat and cold.* Reduce inflammation by applying an ice pack or ice wrapped in a towel for up to 20 minutes several times a day. Or alternate the cold treatment with heat. Try taking a warm shower or using a heating pad on a low setting. Heat can help relax sore muscles, but it sometimes aggravates inflammation, so use it with caution.
- *Rest.* Lie down from time to time to give your neck a rest from holding up your head. Avoid prolonged rest, since too much inactivity can increase stiffness in the neck muscles.
- *Do gentle stretching.* Gently move your neck to one side and hold it for 30 seconds. Stretch your neck in as many directions as the pain allows. This may help alleviate some of the pain.
- *Take frequent breaks.* This is especially helpful if you drive long distances or work long hours at your computer. Keep your head back, over your spine, to reduce strain. Avoid gritting your teeth.
- *Adjust your computer.* Make sure your desk, chair and computer are aligned so the computer monitor is at eye level. When you sit, your knees should be slightly lower than your hips. Use your chair's armrests.
- *Be wise with your phone.* Avoid tucking the phone between your ear and shoulder as you talk. If you use the phone a lot, get a headset.
- *Avoid sleeping on your stomach.* This position puts stress on your neck. Choose a pillow that supports the natural curve of your neck.

Nosebleeds

The lining of your nose contains tiny blood vessels that lie close to the surface and are easily damaged, which may cause bleeding. Most often, nosebleeds are a nuisance and not a true medical problem.

The most common causes of nosebleeds are:
- Dry air — when your nasal membranes are dry, they're more susceptible to bleeding
- Nose picking

Other causes of nosebleeds include sinusitis, allergies, the common cold, a foreign body in the nose, trauma, exposure to chemical irritants, such as ammonia, and taking blood thinners, such as warfarin (Coumadin) and heparin.

Rarely, frequent nosebleeds may indicate a serious condition such as a bleeding disorder or leukemia. See your doctor to rule out these conditions if you experience frequent nosebleeds along with easy bruising and bleeding elsewhere in your body.

Medical help

Seek medical care if:
- You have frequent nosebleeds
- The bleeding lasts for more than 20 minutes and is not slowing
- The bleeding is rapid or the amount of blood loss is great
- Bleeding begins by trickling down the back of your throat
- Other body sites are bruised or bleeding
- The nosebleed follows an accident, a fall or an injury to your head, including trauma that may have broken your nose

Home remedies

To treat a nosebleed:
- Sit upright and lean forward. By remaining upright, you reduce blood pressure in the veins of your nose. This discourages further bleeding. Sitting forward will help you avoid swallowing blood, which can irritate your stomach.
- Pinch the soft part at the bottom of your nose with your thumb and index finger and breathe through your mouth. Continue to pinch for five to 10 minutes. This maneuver puts pressure on the bleeding point and often stops the flow of blood.

To prevent a resumption of bleeding:
- Don't blow your nose or bend down until several hours after the bleeding episode. Keep your head higher than the level of your heart. Don't pick your nose.
- If re-bleeding occurs, gently blow out to clear your nose of blood clots, and spray both nostrils with a decongestant nasal spray containing oxymetazoline (Afrin, others) or phenylephrine (Neo-Synephrine). Pinch your nose again for 10 minutes.

To prevent nosebleeds:
- Increase the humidity of the air you breathe in your home. A humidifier or vaporizer can help keep your nasal membranes moist.
- Over-the-counter saline nasal spray or gel may help, especially during winter months.
- Avoid placing anything in your nose, including tissue, cotton swabs or fingers.

Object in ear

A foreign object becoming stuck in the ear is a relatively common problem. Children, in particular, have a penchant for sticking eraser tips, small toys, dried beans or other pieces of food into their ear canals — they may not know any better or they're simply curious about what will happen.

When an object becomes stuck in the ear, it's important for you and your child to stay calm and assess the situation. There may be some pain and temporary hearing loss but, in general, the object can be safely removed with minimal discomfort.

Medical help

If these methods fail or the person continues to experience pain in the ear, hearing loss or a sensation of something lodged in the ear, seek medical assistance.

Home remedies

If an object becomes lodged in the ear, follow these steps:

- *Don't probe the ear with a tool.* Don't attempt to remove the foreign object by probing with a cotton swab, matchstick or any other tool. To do so is to risk pushing the object farther into the ear and damaging the fragile structures of the middle ear.
- *Remove the object if possible.* If the object is clearly visible, is pliable and can be grasped easily with tweezers, gently remove it.
- *Try using the pull of gravity.* Tilt the head to the affected side. Don't strike the person's head, but shake it gently in the direction of the ground to try to dislodge the object.
- *If the foreign object is an insect, try using oil.* Tilt the person's head so that the ear with the offending insect is turned upward. Try to float the insect out by pouring mineral oil, olive oil or baby oil into the ear. The oil should be warm but not hot. You can ease entry of the oil by straightening the ear canal. Pull the earlobe gently backward and upward. The insect should suffocate and may float out in the oil bath. Don't use oil to remove any object other than an insect. Don't use this method if there's any suspicion of a perforation in the eardrum (pain, bleeding or discharge from the ear).

Object in eye

Most everyone will get a foreign object in an eye at some point. Often, it's a loose eyelash or a dirt speck blown by the wind. The eye often is able to clear itself by tearing up and blinking.

At other times, the eye doesn't clear itself so easily and you may need assistance. On these occasions, follow the guidelines listed on this page.

You may experience minor discomfort, such as a mild scratchy feeling, in the eyeball after the object has been removed. If you continue to feel discomfort after a day or two, seek medical assistance.

If the object is embedded in the eyeball, don't attempt to remove the object and don't rub the eye. Cover both eyes with a soft pad and seek emergency medical care.

Medical help

Seek emergency medical help when:
- You can't remove the object
- The object is embedded in the eyeball
- The person is experiencing abnormal vision
- Pain, vision problems or redness persists

Home remedies

Clearing your own eye
- If it's a minor issue, such as small particles of dust, blinking several times may remove the particles.
- If blinking doesn't work, try to flush the object out of your eye with clean, lukewarm water or saline solution. Use an eyecup or small clean glass. Position the glass with its rim resting on the bone of your eye socket and pour the fluid in, keeping the eye open.

Clearing someone else's eye
- Wash your hands. Seat the person in a well-lighted area.
- Examine the eye to find the object. Gently pull the lower lid down and ask the person to look up. Then hold the upper lid while the person looks down.
- If the object is floating in the tear film or on the surface of the eye, try flushing it out. If you're able to remove the object, flush the eye with a saline solution or clean, lukewarm water.

Don'ts
- Don't rub the eye, and don't apply patches or ice packs to the eye.
- Don't try to remove an object that's embedded in the eyeball.
- Don't try to remove any object that makes closing the eye difficult.

Oral thrush

Oral thrush (candidiasis) is an infection caused by a fungus that accumulates in your mouth. Symptoms may include creamy-white soft patches in your mouth or throat, lesions with a cottage cheese-like appearance, pain, slight bleeding if the lesions are rubbed or scraped, cracking at the corners of your mouth, a cottony feeling in your mouth, or loss of taste.

Oral thrush is most common among babies, young children and older adults. It often occurs when your immune system is weakened by disease or drugs such as prednisone, or when antibiotics disturb the natural balance of microorganisms in your body.

Oral thrush is a minor disorder if you're healthy, but it may be a sign of a weakened immune system. In this case, symptoms may be more severe and harder to control.

Medical help

If you or your baby develops painful white lesions inside the mouth, see your doctor or dentist. If thrush develops in older children or adolescents who have no other risk factors, seek medical care. An underlying condition such as diabetes may be the cause.

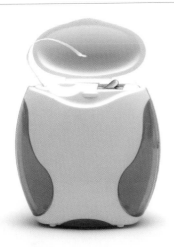

Home remedies

These suggestions may help during an outbreak of oral thrush:

- *Practice good oral hygiene.* Brush at least twice a day and floss at least once. Replace your toothbrush frequently until the infection clears up. Avoid mouthwash or sprays.
- *Try warm saltwater rinses.* Dissolve 1/2 teaspoon of salt in 1 cup of warm water. Swish the rinse and then spit it out, but don't swallow.
- *Keep baby equipment clean.* If your baby develops thrush, clean pacifiers and bottle nipples with a 50 percent vinegar and water solution. If you use a breast pump, use the vinegar solution to clean detachable parts that come in contact with your milk.
- *Use nursing pads.* If you're breast-feeding and develop a fungal infection, this will help prevent the fungus from spreading to your clothes. Look for pads that don't have a plastic barrier, which can encourage growth of the fungus.

Prevention

The following measures may help prevent fungal infections from occurring:

- *Rinse your mouth.* If you have to use a corticosteroid inhaler, be sure to rinse your mouth with water or brush your teeth after taking your medication.
- *Eat yogurt.* Eat fresh-culture yogurt containing *Lactobacillus acidophilus* or *bifidobacterium* or take *acidophilus* capsules when you take antibiotics.
- *Don't ignore vaginal yeast infections.* Treat them immediately.
- *See your dentist regularly — especially if you have diabetes or wear dentures.* Ask your dentist how often you need to schedule a visit. Brush and floss your teeth as often as your dentist recommends. If you wear dentures, be sure to clean them every night.
- *Watch what you eat.* Try limiting the amount of sugar- and yeast-containing foods you consume. These foods may encourage fungal growth.

Osteoporosis

Osteoporosis is a disease that causes your bones to become weak and brittle — so brittle that a minor fall or even mild stress (like bending over or coughing) can fracture a bone. Most of these fractures will occur in the spine, hip or wrist.

Although it's often thought of as a women's disease, osteoporosis affects men as well. And aside from people who have osteoporosis, many others have low bone density that puts them at greater risk of osteoporosis.

To understand osteoporosis, it helps to be aware of the bone remodeling process taking place in your body. Bone continuously changes — new bone is made and old bone is broken down. When you're young, your body builds new bone faster than old bone breaks down.

You generally reach your peak bone mass in your late 20s to early 30s. After that, bone remodeling changes — you begin to lose slightly more bone than you gain. Your likelihood of developing osteoporosis depends on the bone mass you attained by early adulthood, and how rapidly you lose it later.

In the early stages of bone loss, there is usually no indication of a problem. But once your bones are weakened by osteoporosis, signs and symptoms may include:

- Back pain
- Loss of height
- Stooped posture
- Fracture of the vertebra, wrist, hip or other bone

Risk factors

A diet lacking in calcium, phosphorus and other minerals (along with vitamin D) is a critical factor in the development of osteoporosis. If your bones have too little of these minerals, they become weak and brittle. You'll have a lower peak bone mass and accelerated bone loss later in life.

A number of other factors increase the likelihood that you'll develop osteoporosis. They include:

- Being female
- Getting older
- Having a family history of the disease
- Being of Caucasian or Asian descent
- Having a small body frame

Other risk factors include being inactive, tobacco use, having an eating disorder, excessive alcohol consumption and the use of certain medications such as corticosteroids.

Daily calcium

The 2015-2020 Dietary Guidelines for Americans lists the following recommended dietary allowances (RDAs) for calcium:

- Ages 1 to 3 years — 700 mg
- Ages 4 to 8 years — 1,000 mg
- Ages 9 to 18 years — 1,300 mg
- Ages 19 to 50 years — 1,000 mg
- Age 51 to 70 years — 1,000 mg (men) or 1,200 (women)
- Age 71 and older — 1,200 mg

Medical help

Because osteoporosis rarely causes signs and symptoms until it's advanced, bone density testing is recommended if you are:

- A woman older than age 65 or a man older than age 70, regardless of risk factors
- A postmenopausal woman with at least one risk factor
- A man between ages 50 and 70 who has at least one risk factor
- Older than age 50 with a history of a broken bone
- A man or woman and take medications, such as prednisone, aromatase inhibitors or anti-seizure drugs
- A postmenopausal woman who has recently stopped taking hormone therapy
- A woman who experienced early menopause

Home remedies

The following suggestions may help relieve symptoms and prevent osteoporosis:

Posture

Good posture puts less stress on your spine. When you sit or drive, place a rolled towel in the small of your back. Don't lean over while reading or doing handwork. When lifting, bend at your knees, not your waist, and lift with your legs, keeping your upper back straight.

Calcium

See the table on page 138 for recommendations for daily amounts of calcium in your diet.

Dairy products are one, but by no means the only, source of calcium. Almonds, broccoli, spinach, cooked kale, canned salmon with the bones, sardines and soy products, such as tofu and tempeh, also are rich in calcium.

If you find it difficult to get enough calcium, consider taking calcium supplements. The Institute of Medicine recommends taking no more than 2,500 mg of calcium daily.

Vitamin D

Getting adequate amounts of vitamin D is just as important as calcium. Scientists don't yet know the optimal daily dose of vitamin D, but experts generally recommend that adults get between 800 and 1,200 international units (IUs) daily.

Many people get enough vitamin D from sunlight, but this may not be a good source for everyone. Although vitamin D is present in oily fish, such as tuna and sardines, and in egg yolks, you probably don't eat these on a daily basis. Vitamin D supplements are a good alternative.

Exercise

Exercise will benefit your bones no matter at what age you start, but you'll gain the most benefits if you start exercising regularly when you're young and continue to exercise throughout your life.

Combine strength training with weight-bearing exercises. Strength training will help strengthen your arms and upper spine. Weight-bearing exercises, such as walking, jogging, stair climbing, skipping rope, skiing and impact-producing sports, mainly affect your legs, hips and lower spine.

Don't smoke

Smoking may increase bone loss.

Avoid excessive alcohol

Drinking more than two alcoholic drinks daily may decrease bone formation and reduce your body's ability to absorb calcium.

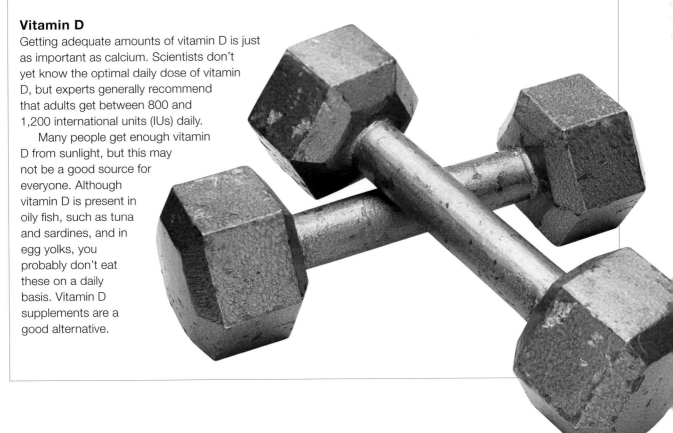

Pink eye

Pink eye, also known as conjunctivitis, is an inflammation or infection of the transparent membrane lining your eyeball. The inflammation causes small blood vessels in the membrane to become more prominent, causing the whites of your eyes to take on a pink or red color.

The condition generally results from a virus or bacteria. Sometimes, it may be due to an allergic reaction. Both viral and bacterial forms are very contagious. Adults and children can develop either type of pink eye, but the bacterial form is more common in children than in adults.

Symptoms of pink eye include redness, itchiness or a gritty feeling in the affected eye, as well as tearing and discharge, blurred vision, and sensitivity to light.

Eyedrops or ointment prescribed by a doctor can treat bacterial pink eye, but there's no treatment for the viral form. Like the common cold, the condition has to run its course. Pink eye generally remains contagious as long as there's tearing and discharge continues to form on the eye.

Viral or bacterial?

You may be able to determine the type of pink eye you have by the discharge.
- **Viral type.** Discharge is usually watery and clear.
- **Bacterial type.** Discharge is often a thick, yellow-green matter.

Home remedies

Take these steps:
- *Apply a warm compress.* Soak a clean, lint-free cloth in warm water, squeeze it dry and place it over your gently closed eyelid. Do this several times daily. In case of allergic conjunctivitis, use a cold compress.
- *Control its spread.* To prevent it from spreading to the other eye or to other people, keep your hands away from your eyes and wash your hands frequently. Also change your washcloth and towel daily. Get rid of eye cosmetics, particularly mascara.
- *Don't wear contacts.* If you wear disposable contacts, throw out your current pair. Disinfect nondisposable types thoroughly. Wait until your eyes are no longer red and you don't have any discharge before wearing contacts again.

Medical help

If you think you may have bacterial conjunctivitis, or you have eye pain or your vision is affected, see your doctor. Also see a doctor if your symptoms worsen.

Poison ivy rash

Contact with the poison ivy plant — or its cousins, poison oak and poison sumac — usually causes red, swollen skin, blisters and severe itching. An oily resin triggers the reaction after direct contact between the plant and your skin, but the resin can transfer easily to skin from exposed clothing or pet hair.

Poison ivy rash typically develops within 12 to 48 hours after exposure. Its severity depends on the amount of resin that gets on your skin. Symptoms usually last for a week or two, but may last longer in people who are more sensitive to poison ivy. Some people experience scarring.

Medical help

If you have a severe reaction, or your eyes, face or genital area is involved, contact your doctor. Also seek medical help if the blisters begin to ooze pus or you develop a fever greater than 100 F.

Home remedies

To reduce signs and symptoms that accompany a poison ivy rash:

- *Wash up quickly.* Washing the poison ivy resin off your skin with soap soon after exposure may avert a skin reaction. Be sure to wash under your fingernails. Don't take a bath — this can spread the resin to other parts of your body.
- *Try not to scratch.* Once the rash has broken out, over-the-counter products such as corticosteroid creams, calamine lotion or creams containing menthol can help ease itching.
- *Cool the itch.* Place cool, wet compresses on the rash for 15 to 30 minutes several times a day. Cool-water tub soaks with baking soda (1/2 to 1 cup) or colloidal oatmeal (Aveeno) also may help.
- *Prevent infection.* Cover open blisters with sterile gauze.
- *Try antihistamines at night.* Oral antihistamines may help you sleep better at night.

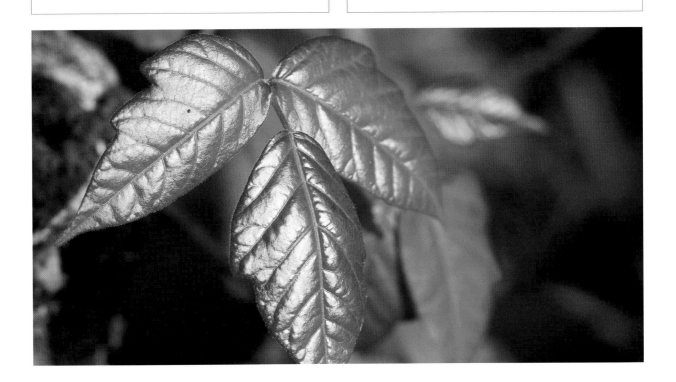

Premenstrual syndrome (PMS)

If you routinely experience a wide variety of physical and emotional changes in the days before your period, you may have premenstrual syndrome (PMS). The signs and symptoms tend to recur in a predictable pattern each month, but may be particularly intense in some months and only slightly noticeable in others.

The condition is related to normal hormone cycles and occurs with normal hormone levels. For most women, signs and symptoms disappear as the menstrual period begins, but for some, the physical pain and emotional stress are severe enough to affect their daily routines and activities.

Exactly what causes premenstrual syndrome is unknown, but several factors may contribute to the condition:

Cyclic changes in hormones

Signs and symptoms occur with regular hormonal fluctuations.

Chemical changes in brain

Fluctuations of certain brain chemicals may trigger symptoms.

Depression and stress

These factors may make signs and symptoms more severe.

Poor eating habits

Some symptoms of PMS are linked to low levels of vitamins and minerals. Eating salty foods and drinking alcoholic or caffeinated beverages may also intensify certain symptoms.

PMS symptoms

Although the list of potential signs and symptoms is long, most women with premenstrual syndrome experience only a few of these problems.

Emotional changes
- Depressed mood and crying spells
- Irritability or anger
- Tension or anxiety
- Mood swings
- Poor concentration
- Lethargy
- Appetite changes and food cravings
- Trouble falling asleep
- Social withdrawal

Physical changes
- Abdominal bloating
- Weight gain from fluid retention
- Swollen hands and feet
- Breast tenderness
- Headache
- Acne flare-ups
- Joint or muscle pain
- Diarrhea or constipation
- Fatigue, nausea and vomiting

Medical help

If you've had no luck managing premenstrual syndrome with lifestyle changes, and signs and symptoms are seriously affecting your health, mood and daily activities, see your doctor.

Home remedies

You can usually manage PMS with a combination of lifestyle changes.

Modify your diet

The following may reduce symptoms:

- Eat smaller, more frequent meals to reduce bloating and the sensation of fullness.
- Limit salt and salty foods to reduce fluid retention.
- Choose foods high in complex carbohydrates, such as fruits, vegetables and whole grains.
- Choose foods rich in calcium, such as fat-free or low-fat dairy products. If you can't tolerate dairy products or aren't getting adequate calcium in your diet, you might consider taking a daily calcium supplement.
- Avoid caffeine and alcohol.

Exercise regularly

Regular exercise can alleviate many symptoms, such as fatigue. Go for a brisk walk, cycle, swim or do another aerobic activity on most days of the week.

Reduce stress

Stress tends to aggravate the symptoms of PMS.

- Plan ahead for PMS. Don't overbook yourself during the week that you're expecting symptoms to occur.
- Get plenty of sleep.
- Practice various types of relaxation therapy. Progressive muscle relaxation or deep-breathing exercises can help reduce headaches, anxiety or insomnia. Consider yoga, tai chi or meditation.

Take supplements

The following supplements may help improve your PMS symptoms:

- *Calcium.* Consuming 1,000 to 1,200 milligrams (mg) of dietary or supplemental calcium daily, such as chewable calcium carbonate (Tums, Rolaids, others), may reduce some symptoms of PMS. Regular use of calcium carbonate also reduces your risk of osteoporosis.
- *Vitamin D.* Research suggests that a high intake of calcium and vitamin D may reduce a woman's risk of PMS.
- *Magnesium.* Taking 400 mg of supplemental magnesium daily may help to reduce fluid retention, breast tenderness and bloating in women with premenstrual syndrome.

Record your symptoms

Keeping a record for a few months may help identify the triggers and timing of your symptoms. You may find that PMS is more tolerable if you see that your symptoms are predictable and short-lived.

Psoriasis

Psoriasis is a disease that causes cells to build up rapidly on the surface of the skin, forming thick silvery scales and itchy, dry red patches. The patches can range from small spots of dandruff-like scaling to major eruptions over large areas of your body. The knees, elbows, trunk and scalp are common locations.

Mild cases of psoriasis may be a nuisance, but more-severe cases can be painful, disfiguring and disabling. Most types of psoriasis go through cycles, flaring for a few weeks or months, and then subsiding or even going into complete remission. Usually, however, the disease returns.

Psoriasis isn't contagious — you can't spread it to other parts of your own body, or to other people, via touch. Factors that may trigger a flare-up include certain types of infections, skin injuries — such as cuts, scrapes or bug bites — stress, cold weather and smoking.

Medical help

If you suspect that you may have psoriasis, see your doctor for a complete examination. Also, talk to your doctor if your psoriasis:

- Progresses beyond the nuisance stage, causing discomfort
- Makes performing routine tasks difficult
- Causes you concern about the appearance of your skin

If you have psoriasis, it's also important to be screened for other conditions that can be associated with psoriasis, including inflammatory bowel disease and inflammatory arthritis.

Home remedies

These measures won't cure psoriasis, but they may help improve the appearance and feel of damaged skin:

- *Take daily baths.* Bathing daily helps remove scales and calm inflamed skin. Use lukewarm water and mild soaps that have added oils and fats. Add bath oil, colloidal oatmeal or Epsom salts to the water and soak for at least 15 minutes.
- *Use moisturizer.* Blot your skin after bathing, then immediately apply a heavy, ointment-based moisturizer while your skin is still moist. For very dry skin, oils may be preferable. During cold, dry weather, you may need to apply moisturizer several times a day.
- *Cover the affected areas overnight.* Apply an ointment-based moisturizer to your skin and wrap with plastic wrap overnight. In the morning, remove the covering and wash away scales.
- *Expose your skin to small amounts of sunlight.* Exposing affected skin to short sessions of sunlight three or more times a week can improve lesions. Too much sun can trigger or worsen outbreaks and increase the risk of skin cancer. Be sure to protect healthy skin with sunscreen with a sun protection factor (SPF) of at least 30.
- *Apply medicated cream or ointment.* Apply an over-the-counter cream or ointment containing hydrocortisone or salicylic acid to reduce itching and scaling. If you have scalp psoriasis, try a medicated shampoo that contains coal tar.
- *Avoid psoriasis triggers, if possible.* Find out what may trigger your psoriasis and take steps to avoid it.
- *Avoid drinking alcohol.* Alcohol consumption may decrease the effectiveness of some psoriasis treatments.

Raynaud's disease

Raynaud's disease is a condition that causes some areas of your body — such as your fingers, toes, ears and tip of your nose — to feel numb and cool in response to cold temperatures or stress. The small arteries that supply blood to your skin temporarily become narrower, limiting blood circulation to the affected areas.

Women are more likely to have Raynaud's disease than are men. It's also more common in people living in colder climates.

Raynaud's disease is more than simply having cold fingers and toes. Signs and symptoms also include:

- A sequence of color changes in your skin in response to the cold or stress
- Numb, prickly feeling or stinging pain as your skin warms or the stress ends

A flare-up may last from less than a minute up to several hours. The affected areas feel cold and numb, usually turning white, then blue, and then red. As circulation improves, the affected areas throb, tingle or swell. Not everyone experiences symptoms in the same sequence.

Medical help

See your doctor right away if you have a history of severe Raynaud's flare-ups and develop an ulcer or infection in one of your affected fingers or toes.

Home remedies

These steps can decrease flare-ups and help you feel better:

- *Don't smoke.* Smoking constricts your blood vessels, causing skin temperature to drop, which may trigger an attack.
- *Exercise.* Regular exercise helps increase blood circulation.
- *Control stress.* Because stress may trigger an attack, learning to avoid stressful situations may help control the disease.
- *Avoid caffeine.* Caffeine products cause your blood vessels to narrow and may increase the signs and symptoms of Raynaud's disease.
- *Take care of your hands and feet.* If you have Raynaud's, guard your hands and feet from injury. Avoid wearing anything that compresses the blood vessels in your hands or feet, such as tight wristbands, rings or footwear.
- *Try niacin.* Niacin, also known as vitamin B-3, causes blood vessels to dilate, increasing blood flow to skin. Niacin supplements may be useful in treating Raynaud's disease, although they may have side effects.
- *Don't take certain medications.* Avoid medications or substances that cause blood vessels to narrow, such as phenylephrine, pseudoephedrine, amphetamine, ergotamine and ephedra.

During flare-ups

If you're experiencing a flare-up of Raynaud's disease, your priority is to warm the affected area. To gently warm your fingers and toes:

- Move to a warmer area.
- Place your hands under your armpits.
- Wiggle your fingers and toes.
- Run warm — not hot — water over your fingers and toes.
- Massage your hands and feet.

Restless legs syndrome

Restless legs syndrome (RLS) is a condition in which your legs feel extremely uncomfortable while you're still. People typically describe the unpleasant sensation as crawling, tingling, electric, itchy or aching. When this occurs, you struggle with uncontrollable urges to move around.

The condition can begin at any age and generally worsens as you get older. Women are more likely than men to develop it. RLS can disrupt sleep — leading to daytime drowsiness — and makes traveling very difficult.

Characteristic features of restless legs syndrome include:

- Symptoms start after you've been sitting or lying down for an extended period of time.
- Movement relieves symptoms — at least temporarily.
- Symptoms are typically better during the day and worsen in the evening.
- There's an association with a condition called periodic limb movements of sleep (PLMS), which causes you to involuntarily flex and extend your legs while sleeping.

Medical help

Some people with RLS never seek medical attention because they worry that their symptoms are too difficult to describe or won't be taken seriously. However, if you think you may have RLS or if the remedies at right don't improve your symptoms, see your doctor.

Home remedies

Simple lifestyle changes can play an important role in helping you alleviate signs and symptoms of RLS:

- *Take pain relievers.* Over-the-counter pain relievers such as ibuprofen (Advil, Motrin IB, others) may relieve mild symptoms.
- *Try baths and massages.* Soaking in a warm bath and massaging your legs can relax your muscles.
- *Apply warm or cool packs.* The use of heat or cold, or alternating use of the two, may lessen the sensations in your limbs.
- *Try relaxation techniques, such as meditation or yoga.*
- *Establish good sleep habits.* Fatigue tends to worsen symptoms of RLS. Create a cool, quiet and comfortable sleeping environment, going to bed at the same time, rising at the same time, and getting enough sleep to feel well-rested.
- *Exercise.* Moderate, regular exercise may relieve symptoms of RLS, but overdoing it at the gym may intensify symptoms.
- *Avoid caffeine.* Sometimes cutting back on caffeine-containing products may help relieve your symptoms.
- *Cut back on alcohol and tobacco.* These substances may aggravate or trigger symptoms. Test to see whether avoiding them helps.

Shin splints

The term shin splints refers to pain along the shinbone (tibia), the large bone in the front of your lower leg. The pain is caused by inflammation in the bone and where the muscles attach to bone.

Shin splints are associated with athletic activity and typically a result of overuse — training too hard, too fast or for too long. It commonly occurs with runners, basketball players, tennis players and army recruits.

If you develop shin splints, you may notice:
- Tenderness, soreness or pain along the inner part of your lower leg
- Mild swelling

At first, the pain may stop when you stop running or exercising. Eventually, however, the pain may become continuous.

Medical help

Seek prompt medical care if:
- Severe pain in your shin follows a fall or accident
- Your shin is red and inflamed
- Shin pain persists at rest, at night or with walking

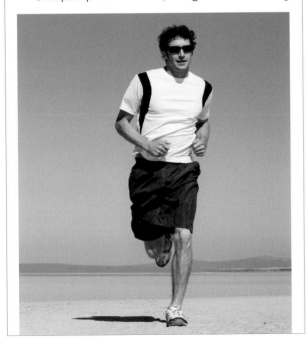

Home remedies

In most cases, you can treat shin splints with simple self-care steps:
- *Rest.* Avoid activities that cause pain, swelling or discomfort — but don't give up all activity. While you're healing, try low-impact exercises, such as swimming or bicycling. If pain causes you to limp, consider using crutches until you can walk normally.
- *Ice the affected area.* Apply ice packs for 15 to 20 minutes and four to eight times a day for several days. To protect your skin, wrap the ice packs in a thin towel.
- *Reduce swelling.* Elevate the shin above the level of your heart, especially at night. During the day, it may help to compress the area with an elastic bandage or compression sleeve — but loosen the wrap if the pain increases or the area becomes numb.
- *Take an over-the-counter pain reliever.* Try aspirin, ibuprofen (Advil, Motrin IB, others), naproxen (Aleve) or acetaminophen (Tylenol, others) to reduce pain.
- *Wear proper shoes.* Your doctor may recommend a shoe that's especially suited for your foot type, stride and particular sport.
- *Consider arch supports.* Arch supports can help cushion and disperse stress on your shinbones.
- *Resume usual activities gradually.* Returning to usual activities too soon, before you heal, may cause continued pain and prolong your recovery.

Prevention
- Begin a run with jogging to loosen the muscles in your legs and feet.
- Consider arch supports to prevent shin pain, especially if you have flat feet or high arches.
- Cross-train with a sport that places less impact on your shins, such as swimming, walking or biking.
- Consult a trainer to evaluate and adjust your running style.

Shingles

Shingles (herpes zoster) is a viral infection that causes a painful rash. It's caused by the same virus that causes chickenpox. After you've had chickenpox, the virus lies inactive in nerve tissue near your spinal cord and, years later, may reactivate as shingles.

Pain is usually the first symptom of shingles. For some, the pain can be intense and is sometimes mistaken for a symptom of problems affecting the heart, lungs or kidneys.

A shingles rash usually appears a few days after the pain. It often develops as a band of blisters wrapping around one side of your body from your back to your front. The blisters usually dry up in a few days, forming crusts that fall off over the next few weeks.

While shingles isn't a life-threatening condition, it can be very painful. The blisters contain a contagious virus, so avoid contact with others, especially people with weak immunity, pregnant women and newborns.

Medical help

Contact your doctor if you suspect shingles, especially in the following situations:
- The pain and rash occur near your eyes. If left untreated, this infection can cause permanent eye damage.
- You or someone in your family has a weakened immune system (due to cancer, medications or a chronic medical condition).
- The rash is widespread and painful.

Home remedies

You can relieve some discomfort of shingles with the following:
- Take a cool bath or soak the blisters with cool, wet compresses.
- Apply a lubricating cream or ointment.
- Take over-the-counter pain relievers, such as aspirin, ibuprofen (Advil, Motrin IB, others), naproxen (Aleve) and acetaminophen (Tylenol, others) to alleviate pain.
- Rubbing over-the-counter creams or ointments on your skin to reduce pain also may be helpful.

Prevention

A shingles vaccine is recommended for all adults age 60 and older, whether or not they've had shingles previously. The vaccine is for prevention, not treatment. Getting the vaccine doesn't guarantee that you won't get shingles, but it will likely reduce the course and severity of the disease. It may also reduce your risk of postherpetic neuralgia, a nerve-related chronic pain condition that can follow shingles.

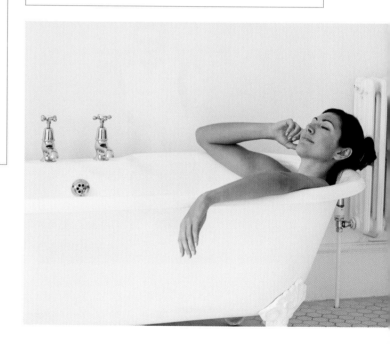

Shoulder pain

Pain can arise from within the shoulder joints and surrounding muscles, ligaments and tendons. The pain usually worsens when you move your arm and shoulder. Pain that doesn't get worse when you move your shoulder is more likely to be "referred pain" caused by a condition or problem in your neck, chest or abdomen.

Bursitis and tendinitis (see pages 35 and 171) are common causes of shoulder pain that occur from overuse. Acute injuries can result in tears to the muscle group that surrounds the shoulder joint (rotator cuff).

Overuse shoulder pain

Shoulder pain that results from overuse centers on the front and outer side of your upper arm. It may be very painful to put on a coat, extend your arm straight out from your side or reach behind you. It also may be uncomfortable to lie on the shoulder at night.

Rotator cuff injury

This type of injury usually results from repetitive overhead motions, such as painting a ceiling, swimming or throwing a baseball, or from trauma, such as falling on your shoulder.

Medical help

Seek medical care if:
- You can't raise the affected arm
- You have extreme tenderness at your collarbone or shoulder
- You have redness, swelling or fever
- Pain isn't improving after a week of self-care

Call 911 if you have shoulder pain accompanied by chest pain, difficulty breathing, cold sweats, feeling faint, or nausea or vomiting

Home remedies

To relieve shoulder pain:
- *Rest your shoulder.* Stop doing what caused the pain. Limit heavy lifting or overhead activity for four to seven days until your shoulder starts to feel better.
- *Apply ice and heat.* Use a cold pack, a bag of frozen vegetables or a towel filled with ice cubes for 15 to 20 minutes at a time to help reduce inflammation. Do this every couple of hours. After two or three days, when the pain and inflammation have improved, hot packs or a heating pad may help relax sore muscles. Limit heat applications to 20 minutes.
- *Use over-the-counter pain medications.* This includes aspirin, ibuprofen (Advil, Motrin IB, others), naproxen (Aleve) and acetaminophen (Tylenol, others). However, seek medical advice if you have any kidney problems or stomach problems before using NSAIDs.
- *Do stretching exercises.* After one or two days, do gentle exercises to keep your shoulder muscles limber. If possible, put the shoulder through its full range of motion. Inactivity can cause stiff joints.
- *Take it slow.* Wait until pain is gone before gradually returning to the activity that caused the injury. This may require three to six weeks.
- *Review your technique.* If an activity — such as a racket sport, baseball, golf or weight training — is involved, you may need to alter your technique.

Sinusitis

Sinusitis occurs when the cavities surrounding your nasal passages (sinuses) become inflamed and swollen. Swelling can close off the passages, making it difficult for the sinuses to drain. Pain may result from the inflammation or from pressure as mucus builds up in the sinus cavities.

Signs and symptoms include pain around your eyes or cheeks, nasal congestion, causing difficulty breathing through your nose, and drainage of a thick, yellow or greenish discharge from the nose or down the back of the throat. There may be aching in your upper jaw and teeth and a reduced sense of taste and smell.

Short-lived (acute) sinusitis is often caused by the common cold. Chronic sinusitis may stem from an infection, allergies, nasal polyps or conditions such as a deviated septum.

Medical help

Contact your doctor if your symptoms don't improve within a few days or they worsen, or if you have a history of recurrent or chronic sinusitis. If your sinusitis is the result of a bacterial infection, your doctor may prescribe an oral antibiotic or other medications.

Home remedies

The following steps can be used to help relieve symptoms of sinusitis:

- *Apply warm compresses.* Place warm, damp towels around your nose, cheeks and eyes to help ease pain.
- *Drink plenty of fluids.* Fluids help dilute nasal secretions and promote drainage. Avoid beverages that contain caffeine or alcohol, because they can be dehydrating. Alcohol can also worsen swelling.
- *Steam your sinuses.* This will ease pain and help mucus to drain. Drape a towel over your head and cautiously inhale steam from a basin of boiling water. Keep the steam directed toward your face. Or take a hot shower, breathing in the warm, moist air.
- *Get plenty of rest.* This will help your body fight infection and speed recovery.
- *Sleep with your head elevated.* This will help your sinuses drain.

Nasal lavage

The rinsing of your nasal passages (lavage) flushes out excess mucus and debris and helps reduce sinus inflammation. Lavage may be performed with a bulb syringe, a specially designed squeeze bottle or a neti pot — a small pot with a long spout, somewhat similar to a teapot. All of these products should be available in pharmacies or medical supply stores.

Fill the squeeze bottle with a mild solution of warm salt water. While standing over a sink, place the tip of the container in one nostril and squeeze, causing the solution to run in that nostril, through your sinuses, and out the other nostril.

With the neti pot, instead of squeezing, pour the solution into a nostril while your head is tipped forward and slightly sideways. As the solution passes through your sinuses, it clears them out.

Beware of decongestant nasal sprays

Decongestant nasal sprays (Afrin, Neo-Synephrine, others) can help open clogged nasal passages, but you should only use them once a day for a short period – up to three days. After a few days of using such a spray, your nasal membranes may become less responsive to the medication and require more spray to alleviate the congestion. When you stop using the spray, your symptoms may become worse — what's known as rebound congestion.

Snoring

Almost half of all adults snore at least occasionally. Snoring occurs when the air you breathe while you're sleeping flows past relaxed tissues in your throat. This causes the tissues to vibrate, creating harsh respiratory sounds.

Depending on its cause, your snoring may be accompanied by restless sleep, gasping or choking at night, a morning headache, excessive daytime sleepiness, a sore throat, high blood pressure, and irregular heartbeats.

Many factors may affect your airway and lead to snoring:

Mouth anatomy

When you doze off, the muscles in roof of your mouth (palate), tongue and throat relax, which can partially obstruct your airway. Having a low, thick palate or enlarged tonsils or tissues in the back of your throat can narrow the airway further and increase the amount of vibration. Being overweight contributes to narrowing of the airway.

Nasal problems

Chronic nasal congestion or a crooked partition between your nostrils (deviated nasal septum) may be to blame for snoring.

Sleep apnea

Snoring may be associated with obstructive sleep apnea, characterized by loud snoring followed by periods of silence that can last for 10 seconds or more. In this serious condition, your airway is obstructed or becomes so small that the amount of air you breathe is inadequate for your needs. Eventually, straining to maintain your breathing against your relaxed throat wakes you up and forces your airway open, accompanied by a loud snort or gasping sound. This pattern may be repeated many times during the night.

Alcohol consumption

Snoring can also be brought on by consuming too much alcohol before bedtime. Alcohol relaxes throat muscles and decreases your natural defenses against airway obstruction.

Medical help

If your snoring doesn't improve, see your doctor. Inform a pediatrician if your child snores. Children, too, can have obstructive sleep apnea, although most don't. Nose and throat problems, such as enlarged tonsils, and obesity often underlie habitual snoring in children. Treating these conditions can help improve sleep.

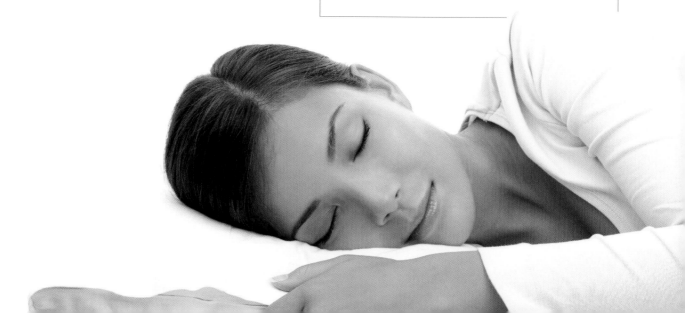

Home remedies

To prevent or ease snoring, try these suggestions:

Lose weight

Being overweight is a common cause of snoring. Extra bulkiness narrows your airway, and loose tissue in your throat is more likely to vibrate as you breathe.

Sleep on your side

Your tongue is more likely to fall backward into your throat when you sleep on your back, which narrows your airway and partially obstructs airflow. To prevent sleeping on your back, try sewing a tennis ball in the back of your pajama top.

Treat nasal congestion

Allergies or a deviated septum can limit airflow through your nose, forcing you to breathe through your mouth and increasing the likelihood of snoring. Don't use decongestants for more than three days in a row for acute congestion unless directed to do so by your doctor. Correcting a deviated septum may require nasal surgery.

Try nasal strips or valves

Another way to keep nasal passages open and reduce breathing through your mouth is with nasal strips, which can be purchased at most drug stores and pharmacies. Attaching the adhesive strips to your nose before bedtime widens the nasal passages, making it easier to breathe and, possibly, reducing snoring, especially if the vibrations originate in your nose.

In addition, adhesive nasal values have been designed to help with snoring by applying gentle pressure to the airways. Nasal valves can be ordered online without a prescription.

Limit or avoid alcohol and sedatives

Avoid alcoholic beverages at least four hours before bedtime. Inform your doctor that you snore before taking sedatives or sleeping pills. These products depress your central nervous system, causing excessive muscle relaxation, including tissues at the base of your throat. Alcohol, sedatives and sleeping pills also blunt your brain's ability to arouse you from sleep. It may take longer for you to start breathing again if you've stopped breathing due to obstructive sleep apnea.

Strengthen your throat muscles

Playing the didgeridoo, a wind instrument that produces a droning sound, may help train your throat muscles and prevent them from narrowing your upper airway. A study from the *British Medical Journal* evaluated use of the instrument by individuals with sleep apnea who complained of snoring. Results show that participants who played the instrument for about 25 minutes a day experienced less daytime sleepiness — a complication of sleep apnea and snoring. However, further study is required.

Get your ZZZs

Sleep deprivation may exaggerate the relaxation of tissues in the back of your throat, producing more snoring. Aim for no less than seven hours of sleep time each night to avoid sleep deprivation.

Sore throat

The tight, scratchy feeling in your throat may be a familiar sign that a cold or flu (influenza) is on the way. Although uncomfortable, most sore throats aren't harmful and go away on their own in five to seven days. Sometimes, you may look to over-the-counter lozenges or gargles for relief.

Most sore throats are caused by viral or bacterial infections. Viruses and bacteria can enter through your mouth or nose — either because you breathe in particles that are released in the air when someone coughs or sneezes, or because you come into physical contact with an infected person or use shared objects such as utensils and tableware, towels, toys, doorknobs, computer keyboards or telephones.

Sore throats can also be caused by allergies and dry air. When a sore throat involves swollen tonsils, it's sometimes called tonsillitis.

Viral infection

Viruses are typically the source of common colds and the flu, and the sore throat that often accompanies them. Colds usually go away once your system has had time to build up antibodies that destroy the virus — which takes about one week. Antibiotic medications can't help in treating viral infections, so don't look to them for fast, effective relief. Recovery takes time.

Common signs and symptoms of viral infection include:
- Sore or scratchy, dry feeling in the throat
- Hoarseness
- Coughing and sneezing
- Runny nose and postnasal dripping
- Mild fever or no fever

Bacterial infection

Bacterial infections aren't as common as viral infections, but they can be more serious. And the most common bacterial cause of throat infection is strep throat. Often, you develop strep throat within two to seven days of being exposed to someone else with the infection. Children ages 5 to 15 in a classroom setting are the most likely to get it.

Streptococcal bacteria — the cause of strep throat — are highly contagious. They can spread by airborne droplets from a cough or sneeze, or through shared food or drinks. You can also pick up the bacteria from a doorknob or other surface and transfer them to your nose or mouth.

Strep throat, if left untreated, can lead to complications such as kidney inflammation (glomerulonephritis) or rheumatic fever. Strep throat requires medical treatment with antibiotics and pain relievers.

Common signs and symptoms of strep throat include:
- Inflamed, swollen tonsils and lymph nodes
- Pain when swallowing
- Bright red color with white patches in the throat
- Fever, generally more than 101 F, and often accompanied by chills

Medical help

Seek emergency care if your sore throat is accompanied by any of the following symptoms:
- Drooling
- Difficulty or pain on swallowing or breathing
- Stiff, rigid neck and severe headache
- Temperature higher than 101 F in babies under age 6 months
- Rash
- Persistent hoarseness or mouth ulcers lasting two weeks or more

Home remedies

Until your sore throat has run its course, try these tips:

- *Double your fluid intake.* Fluids such as water, juice, tea and warm soup help keep your mucus thin and easy to clear. Avoid caffeine and alcohol, which can dehydrate you.
- *Gargle with warm salt water.* Mix about 1/2 teaspoon of salt in a full glass of warm water and gargle. This helps soothe your throat and clear it of mucus.
- *Suck on a lozenge or hard candy.* Chewing sugarless gum also helps. These actions stimulate saliva production, which bathes and cleanses your throat.
- *Drink honey mixed with warm tea or warm lemon water.* This is a time-honored method for soothing a sore throat. Due to the risk of infant botulism, a rare form of food poisoning, never give honey to a child younger than age 1.
- *Take pain relievers.* Over-the-counter medications, such as acetaminophen (Tylenol, others), ibuprofen (Advil, Motrin IB, others) and aspirin, relieve sore throat pain for four to six hours. Don't give aspirin to children or teenagers.

- *Rest your voice.* If a sore throat affects your voice box (larynx), talking may lead to more irritation and temporary loss of your voice — a condition known as laryngitis. Talking as little as possible may help avoid this.
- *Humidify the air.* Adding moisture to the air prevents the mucous membranes in your sinuses and throat from drying out. This can reduce irritation and promote sleep. Saline nasal sprays also are helpful.
- *Avoid smoke and other air pollutants.* Smoke irritates a sore throat. Stop smoking and avoid environmental smoke, as well as fumes from household products. Keep children away from secondhand smoke.

Prevention

To prevent sore throats, follow some age-old advice:

- Wash your hands frequently or use an alcohol-based hand cleanser, especially during the cold and flu seasons.
- Keep your hands away from your face to avoid getting bacteria and viruses into your mouth or nose.

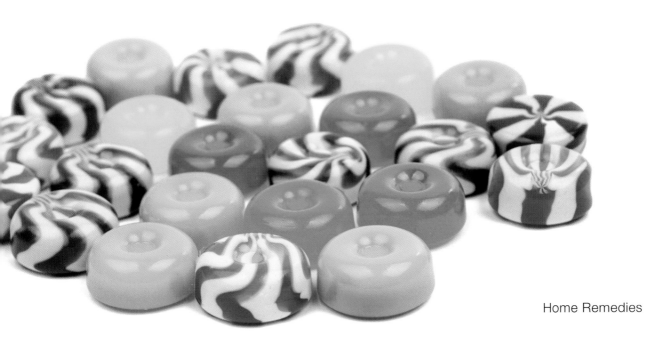

Sprains

Strictly speaking, a sprain occurs whenever you overextend or tear one of your ligaments. Ligaments are the tough, elastic-like bands that connect bone to bone and hold your joints in place. Joint movement that is excessive or beyond normal range — perhaps a violent twist — can tear a ligament partially or completely.

Sprains occur most often in your ankles, knees or the arches of your feet. True sprains are painful and cause rapid swelling. Generally, the greater the pain, the more severe the injury. The severity of a sprain can be:

- **Mild.** A ligament is stretched excessively or tears slightly. The area is tender and somewhat painful, especially with movement. There's not a lot of swelling. You can put weight on the joint.
- **Moderate.** Some fibers are torn but the ligament doesn't rupture completely. The joint is tender, painful and difficult to move. The area may be swollen and discolored from bleeding.
- **Severe.** One or more ligaments tear completely. The area is painful, very swollen and discolored. You're unable to move the joint normally or put any weight on it. The injury may be difficult to distinguish from a fracture or dislocation, both of which require medical care. You may need a cast to hold the joint motionless, or surgery, if the tears cause joint instability.

Preventing sports injuries

To reduce your risk of sprains, strains and other ligament and muscle injuries:

- *Warm up.* Loosen and stretch your muscles at the start of exercise, and gradually increase your level of activity over five to 10 minutes. If you're prone to muscle pain, apply heat before you exercise.
- *Cool down.* After exercising, ease up gradually with muscle stretches. This may help reduce muscle injury and stiffness.
- *Begin gradually.* If you're trying out a new sport, increase your level of exertion in stages over several weeks.
- *Do cross-training.* Combining two or more types of physical activity helps avoid injuries from repetitive stress. You can try multiple activities in the same workout or alternate activities from one day to the next.
- *Don't overdo it.* Stop an activity immediately if you experience chest pain, an irregular heartbeat, dizziness or faintness, pain in an arm or jaw, severe shortness of breath, excessive fatigue, severe joint or muscle pain, or joint swelling.

Medical help

Seek medical care immediately if:

- You hear a popping sound when the injury occurs and you can't use the joint. If possible, apply cold immediately.
- You have a fever and the area is red and hot.
- You have a severe sprain, as described above. Delayed treatment may cause long-term joint instability or chronic pain.

See your doctor if you're unable to bear weight on the joint after two to three days of self-care or if you don't experience much improvement after about a week.

Home remedies

To treat a sprain:
- Follow the instructions for P.R.I.C.E. provided on this page.
- Use over-the-counter pain medications, if needed. Don't exceed the recommended dose unless your doctor advises it.
- After 48 hours, if the swelling is gone, apply gentle heat to the area. Heat can improve blood flow and speed healing.
- Gradually test the injured joint and, if possible, try to use the joint after two days have passed. Mild to moderate sprains usually improve significantly in about one week, although full healing may take up to six weeks.
- Avoid activities that continue to put stress on your injured joint. Repeated minor sprains further weaken the joint.
- Apply cold to sore areas after a workout, even if you're not injured, to prevent inflammation and swelling.

P.R.I.C.E.

You'll see the term *P.R.I.C.E.* mentioned frequently in this book. P.R.I.C.E. is common practice for treating sprained ligaments, muscle strains and joint injuries. The letters stand for Protection, Rest, Ice, Compress and Elevate — actions you take in a sequence to promote healing and help prevent further tissue damage.

- **P:** Protect the area to prevent further injury. You may need to limit or avoid weight-bearing activity or immobilize the area with a splint or brace.
- **R:** Rest the area to promote tissue healing. Avoid activities that cause more pain, swelling or discomfort.
- **I:** Ice the area immediately, even if you seek medical help. Apply an ice pack or immerse the injury in an icy slush bath for 15 minutes. Repeat every two to three hours during waking hours for the first two to three days. Cold reduces swelling and inflammation and may also slow bleeding if a muscle or ligament tear has occurred.
- **C:** Compress the area with an elastic bandage until the swelling stops. Don't wrap it tightly or you may hinder circulation. Begin wrapping at the end farthest from your heart. Loosen the wrap if pain increases, if the area becomes numb or if there is swelling below the wrapped area.
- **E:** Elevate the injured area above the level of your heart, especially at night. For example, you can prop up an injured ankle on pillows. Gravity helps reduce swelling by draining away excess blood and fluid.

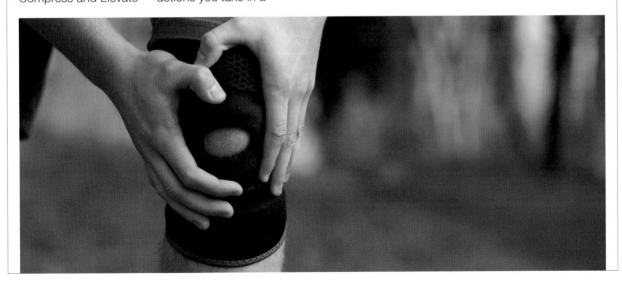

Stomach flu

What people commonly refer to as stomach flu is also known as viral gastroenteritis. This isn't the same thing as influenza. Real flu (influenza) attacks your respiratory system — your nose, throat and lungs. Viral gastroenteritis is an intestinal infection.

Signs and symptoms

Viral gastroenteritis may appear within one to three days after you're infected. Signs and symptoms range from mild to severe, and usually last just a day or two but occasionally persist as long as 10 days. Signs and symptoms typically include:
- Watery, usually nonbloody diarrhea (bloody diarrhea may indicate a different infection)
- Abdominal cramps and pain
- Nausea, vomiting or both
- Occasional muscle ache or headache
- Low-grade fever

Dehydration — a severe loss of water and essential salts and minerals — is a serious complication of stomach flu. For infants, older adults and people with compromised immune systems, stomach flu can be deadly.

Common causes

The ailment is spread through contact with an infected person or from eating or drinking contaminated food or water. In many cases, transmission follows the fecal-oral route — that is, someone with a virus handles food you eat without washing his or her hands after using the bathroom. Different viruses can cause gastroenteritis, including the two most common culprits:

Rotavirus

This virus is the most common cause of infectious diarrhea in children. Children usually are infected when they put fingers or objects contaminated with the virus into their mouths. Infected adults usually don't develop signs and symptoms, but can still spread the illness.

A rotaviral vaccine that's effective in preventing severe symptoms of gastroenteritis is available. Talk to your doctor about whether it's advisable to immunize your child.

Noroviruses

There are several different strains of norovirus, all of which cause similar signs and symptoms. In addition to diarrhea, nausea and vomiting, you may experience muscle ache, a headache, fatigue and a low-grade fever.

A norovirus infection may sweep through families, communities or large groups traveling, for example, on cruise ships. Most often, you pick up the infection from contaminated food or water, but person-to-person transmission also is possible.

After exposure to the virus, you're likely to feel sick within 18 to 72 hours. Most people feel better in a day or two, but you're still contagious for at least three days — and up to two weeks — after recovery.

Signs of dehydration

A serious complication of stomach flu is dehydration. Signs and symptoms include:
- Excessive thirst
- Dry mouth
- Deep yellow urine or little or no urine
- Severe weakness, dizziness, lightheadedness or confusion

Medical help

If you're an adult, call your doctor if:
- You're not able to keep liquids down for 24 hours
- You've been vomiting for more than two days
- You're vomiting blood or have blood in your bowel movements
- You're dehydrated
- You have a fever above 104 F

Call your doctor if your child:
- Has a fever of 102 F or higher that lasts longer than one day (ages 6 to 24 months) or longer than three days (ages 2 and older)

- Seems lethargic or very irritable
- Is in a lot of discomfort or pain
- Has bloody diarrhea
- Seems dehydrated — watch for signs of dehydration by comparing how much they drink and urinate with their normal habits. For infants and children wearing diapers, a good guideline is a minimum of three wet diapers in a 24-hour period.

If you have an infant, remember that spitting up may be an everyday occurrence for your baby, but vomiting is not. Babies vomit for a variety of reasons, many of which may require medical attention.

Home remedies

Keep yourself comfortable and prevent dehydration while you recover with the following steps:
- *Allow your stomach to settle.* No eating for a few hours after vomiting or diarrhea.
- *Suck on ice chips or take small sips of water.* Try to drink plenty of liquid every day, taking small, frequent sips. Also consider clear sodas, clear broths or noncaffeinated sports drinks.
- *Ease back into eating.* Gradually begin eating bland, easy-to-digest foods such as crackers, toast, gelatin, bananas, rice and chicken.
- *Avoid certain foods and beverages.* These include dairy products, caffeine, alcohol, nicotine, and fatty or highly seasoned foods.
- *Get plenty of rest.*
- *Be cautious with medications.* Use medications such as ibuprofen (Advil, Motrin IB, others) sparingly, if at all. They can upset your stomach more. Also be cautious with acetaminophen (Tylenol, others), which can cause liver toxicity.

Treating children
If your child has an intestinal infection, your most important goal is to replace lost fluids and salts.

- *Help your child rehydrate.* Let your child's stomach settle for 15 to 20 minutes after any vomiting or diarrhea occurs, then offer small amounts of liquid. It's best to use oral rehydration solutions such as Pedialyte. In children with gastroenteritis, water isn't absorbed well and doesn't adequately replace lost electrolytes. Avoid giving apple juice — it can make diarrhea worse. If you're breast-feeding, let your baby nurse. If bottle-feeding, offer oral rehydration solution or regular formula.
- *Get back to a normal diet slowly.* Gradually introduce bland, easy-to-digest foods, such as rice, crackers, gelatin and bananas.
- *Avoid certain foods.* Dairy products and sugary foods, such as sodas and candy, can make diarrhea worse.
- *Make sure your child gets plenty of rest.*
- *Be cautious with medications.* Giving a child or teenager aspirin may cause Reye's syndrome, a rare but potentially fatal disease. Avoid giving your child over-the-counter anti-diarrheal medications such as Imodium unless advised by your doctor. They can make it harder for your child's body to eliminate the virus.

Food poisoning culprits

Many bacterial, viral or parasitic agents cause food poisoning, a common cause of stomach flu. This table shows some of the possible contaminants, when you might start to feel symptoms and common ways the organism spreads.

Contaminant	Onset of symptoms	Foods affected and means of transmission
Campylobacter	2 to 5 days	Meat and poultry. Contamination occurs during processing if animal feces come in contact with the meat. Can also spread via unpasteurized milk and contaminated water.
Clostridium perfringens	8 to 16 hours	Meats, stews and gravies. Commonly spread when serving dishes don't keep food hot enough or the food is chilled too slowly.
Escherichia coli (E. coli) O157:H7	1 to 8 days	Beef contaminated during slaughter. Spread mainly by undercooked ground beef. Other sources include unpasteurized milk and apple cider, alfalfa sprouts, and contaminated water.
Giardia lamblia	1 to 2 weeks	Raw, ready-to-eat produce and contaminated water. Can be spread by an infected food handler.
Hepatitis A	28 days	Raw, ready-to-eat produce and shellfish from contaminated water. Can be spread by an infected food handler.
Listeria	9 to 48 hours	Hot dogs, luncheon meats, unpasteurized milk and cheeses, and unwashed raw produce. Can be spread through contaminated soil and water.
Noroviruses (Norwalk-like viruses)	12 to 48 hours	Raw, ready-to-eat produce and shellfish from contaminated water. Can be spread by an infected food handler.
Rotavirus	1 to 3 days	Raw, ready-to-eat produce. Can be spread by an infected food handler.
Salmonella	1 to 3 days	Raw or contaminated meat, poultry, milk or egg yolks. Survives inadequate cooking. Can be spread by knives, cutting surfaces or an infected food handler.
Shigella	24 to 48 hours	Raw, ready-to-eat produce. Can be spread by an infected food handler.
Staphylococcus aureus	1 to 6 hours	Meats and prepared salads, cream sauces and cream-filled pastries. Can be spread by hand contact, coughing and sneezing.
Vibrio vulnificus	1 to 7 days	Raw oysters and raw or undercooked mussels, clams and whole scallops. Can be spread through contaminated seawater.

Limit your risk of illness from these contaminants by:
- Washing hands well before preparing foods
- Keeping raw meat separate from other foods during food preparation
- Cooking meat to the recommended internal temperature
- Refrigerating food within two hours of cooking (or within one hour if room temperature is above 90 F)

Stress and anxiety

Stress is something that just about everyone knows well and experiences often. It's that feeling of pressure, typically a result of too much to do and too little time to do it in. In a busy life, stress is almost unavoidable.

Stress is caused by events that are positive — new job, vacation or marriage — as well as negative — job loss, divorce or death in the family. Stress is not the event itself, but rather your psychological or physical reaction to the event.

Anxiety is a tense feeling that often accompanies stress. It's typically directed toward the future — toward something that may happen soon. Some anxiety can motivate you or help you respond to danger. However, if you have ongoing anxiety that interferes with daily activities and makes it hard to enjoy life, then anxiety can be a problem.

When you experience stress and anxiety, especially if they're severe, your body will respond physically to the threat. Your heart beats faster and breathing quickens. Your blood pressure and blood sugar level rise. Blood flow to your brain and large muscles also increases. After the threat passes, your body slowly relaxes and functions return to normal.

You can usually handle the negative effects of stress when it's occasional, but when stress happens regularly, the effects tend to increase and multiply. Chronic stress is often involved with situations that aren't easily resolved, such as relationship problems, loneliness, financial worries, legal difficulties or long workdays.

Signs and symptoms

Stress and anxiety can produce a variety of physical, emotional and behavioral signs and symptoms.

The earliest indications that your body is feeling under stress may include a headache, upset stomach, diarrhea, constipation and insomnia. A nervous habit such as nail biting may reappear. You may become irritable with people who are close to you.

Occasionally, this response is so gradual that you, your family and friends don't recognize that there's a problem until your health or relationships change.

Sometimes, the signs and symptoms of stress can lead to illness — perhaps aggravating an existing health problem or possibly triggering a new one, if you're already at risk for that condition.

Controlling stress

Learning strategies to manage stress can help reset your body's response to stressful times. Without these tools, your body may remain on high alert, which, over time, can produce serious health problems. Simple strategies are described on page 162.

Medical help

Contact a doctor or mental health professional if stress feels overwhelming or you're unable to function well, physically or emotionally.

Home remedies

To help control stress and anxiety, follow these suggestions:

- *Learn to relax.* The relaxation therapies described here may help you cope with the physical signs and symptoms. Your goal is to lower your heart rate and blood pressure while also reducing muscle tension.
- *Discuss your concerns.* Talking with a trusted friend helps relieve stress and may provide a more positive perspective on your situation. This may lead to a healthy plan of action.
- *Get plenty of sleep.* A healthy body promotes mental health. Sleep provides more vigor and a refreshed state of mind for tackling life's challenges.
- *Stay physically active.* Exercise keeps your body healthy and helps burn off excess energy that stress can produce. Aim for at least 30 minutes of daily exercise. Even brief periods of activity can help reduce tension and improve your mood.
- *Eat regular, balanced meals and healthy snacks.*
- *Limit caffeine.* Too much coffee, tea or soda can increase your level of stress.
- *Plan ahead.* Approach daily responsibilities in a practical and organized fashion. Divide big jobs into smaller tasks and take them on, one task at a time, until you reach your goal.
- *Deal with anger.* Anger can and should be expressed, when it's done carefully. First, count to 10 and compose yourself. Then, respond to strong emotions.
- *Be realistic.* Set goals you can achieve. Concentrate on what's important. Setting unrealistic goals invites failure.
- *Get away.* A change of pace or change of scene may help you develop a whole new outlook.
- *Avoid self-medication.* At times people rely on medication or alcohol for stress relief. This may lead to dependency.
- *Make time to enjoy life.* Going for walks or to the movies, golfing with friends or getting together for a game of cards helps relieve inner pressures.
- *Nurture your inner spirituality.* Nature, art, music, meditation and prayer, as well as religious services, can help build inner strength and perspective.

- *Develop a support network.* Family members, friends and co-workers whom you can turn to for support may be helpful when coping with stress.

Relaxation techniques are an important part of stress management. Relaxation isn't just about finding quiet time or enjoying a hobby. It's a process that helps you repair the toll that stress takes on your mind and body. Relaxation techniques usually involve refocusing your attention on something calming and increasing awareness of your body.

Relaxation therapy

Relaxation therapy includes many techniques, ranging from paced respiration and deep breathing to meditation and progressive muscle relaxation. Most involve the repetition of a single word, phrase or muscular activity, which allows you to "empty" your mind of external thoughts and stressors.

Massage

A number of studies indicate that massage can help control the signs and symptoms of stress and anxiety by relaxing your muscles and calming your mind.

Yoga

Several studies indicate that regularly practicing yoga may help reduce daily stress and anxiety. Kundalini yoga, a type of yoga that's been studied specifically for anxiety disorder, combines poses and breathing techniques with chanting and meditation.

Aromatherapy

Aromatherapy is the science of using oils from various plants to treat illness and promote health. The oils are often vaporized and inhaled or used in massage. It's believed that compounds in the oils activate certain brain chemicals that have a relaxing effect.

Art and music therapy

You can use drawing, painting, clay and sculpture to express your inner thoughts and emotions when talking about them is difficult. The creation and interpretation of art is thought to be therapeutic. Listening to or playing music also has shown to have calming effects.

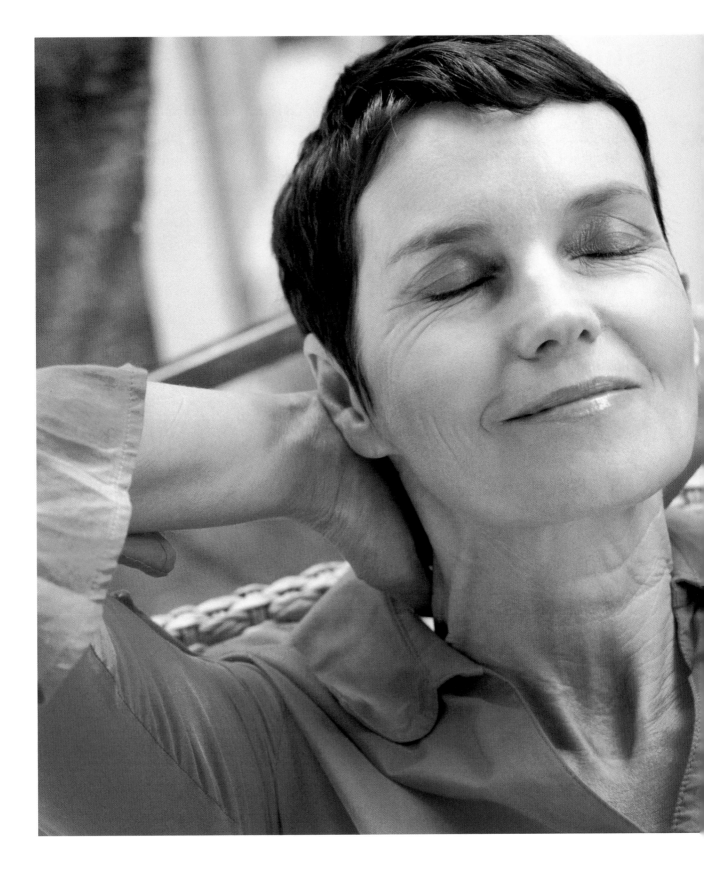

Stuffy nose

A stuffy nose develops when delicate tissue in the nose becomes swollen, often because of blood vessels that are inflamed. The sinus passageways narrow, preventing the easy drainage of mucus and resulting in a "stuffy" feeling. Nasal congestion is just an annoyance for most older children and adults, but it can be serious for infants, who may have a hard time breathing and breast-feeding as a result. The causes of a stuffy nose may include:

- Common cold.
- Obstructions such as nasal polyps, tumors and enlarged adenoids.
- Deformities of the nose and nasal chambers. Deformities such as a deviated septum may result from an injury that occurred years earlier.
- Allergies. Inhaled substances, such as pollen, mold or house dust,can trigger an inflammatory response. This can be seasonal or last year-round.
- Nonallergic rhinitis. Specific triggers such as smoke, air conditioning or vigorous exercise may also cause nasal inflammation.

Medical help

See your doctor if:

- Your symptoms last more than 10 days
- You have a high fever, particularly if it lasts more than three days
- Your nasal discharge is green in color, and accompanied by sinus pain or fever
- You have asthma or emphysema, or you're taking immune-suppressing medications
- You have blood in your nasal discharge or a persistent clear discharge after a head injury

Home remedies

To treat a stuffy nose:

- Gently blow your nose if mucus or debris is present.
- Breathe steam to loosen the mucus and clear your sinuses, or take a warm shower or sit in the bathroom with the shower running.
- Drink plenty of liquids.
- Nonprescription oral decongestants (liquid or pills) may be helpful, but limit nonprescription decongestant nasal sprays or nose drops to no more than three days of use. Taken longer than that, they can make the problem worse.
- Try saline nasal drops or spray or nasal lavage (see page 151). These are safe to use as long as needed.

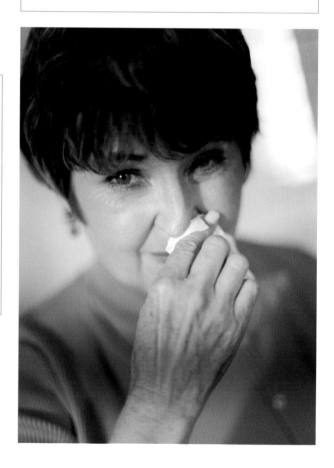

Sunburn

You know a sunburn when it happens: red, painful skin that feels hot to the touch. A sunburn usually appears within a few hours after sun exposure and may take from several days to several weeks to fade. A severe sunburn may include swelling and small fluid-filled blisters. It can also cause a headache, fever and fatigue.

Within a few days, your body starts to heal itself by "peeling" the top layer of damaged skin. After peeling, your skin may temporarily have an irregular color and pattern.

Prevention is best

To protect yourself from a sunburn:
- Try to avoid being outdoors from 10 a.m. to 4 p.m. when the sun's ultraviolet radiation is at its peak.
- Cover exposed areas, wear a broad-brimmed hat and use an ample amount of sunscreen with a sun protection factor (SPF) of at least 30. Reapply sunscreen after swimming and every two hours while out in the sun.
- Protect your eyes. Choose sunglasses that block 99 to 100 percent of ultraviolet rays. For more protection, choose wraparound sunglasses or those that fit close to your face.

Medical help

See your doctor if the sunburn:
- Blisters and covers a large portion of your body
- Is accompanied by a high fever, extreme pain, confusion or nausea
- Doesn't respond to self-care within a few days

Also, seek medical care if you notice:
- Increasing pain, tenderness or swelling
- Yellow drainage (pus) from an open blister
- Red streaks, leading away from the open blister, which may extend in a line upward along the arm or leg

Home remedies

Once a sunburn occurs, you can't do much to limit skin damage. However, the following tips may reduce your pain and discomfort:
- *Take anti-inflammatory medication.* Take aspirin, ibuprofen (Advil, Motrin IB, others) or naproxen (Aleve) until redness and soreness subside. Aspirin isn't recommended for children or teens.
- *Apply cold compresses.* Apply a towel dampened with cool tap water to the affected skin. Or take a cool bath or shower.
- *Apply moisturizers.* A moisturizing cream, aloe vera lotion or low dose (0.5 percent to 1 percent) hydrocortisone cream may decrease pain and swelling, and speed up healing.
- *If blisters form, don't break them.* Blisters form a protective layer to damaged skin. Breaking them slows the healing process and increases the risk of infection. If needed, lightly cover blisters with gauze. If blisters break on their own, apply an antibacterial cream.
- *Drink plenty of fluids.* Exposure to sun and heat causes fluid loss through your skin. Be sure to replenish those fluids to prevent dehydration — when your body doesn't have enough water and other fluids to carry out normal functions.
- *Treat peeling skin gently.* Peeling is simply your body's way of getting rid of the top layer of damaged skin. While your skin is peeling, continue to use moisturizing cream.
- *Beware of topical '-caine' products.* Some of these products, such as benzocaine, claim to relieve sunburn pain. But some dermatologists warn against using such products because they can irritate the skin or cause an allergic reaction.

Sweating and body odor

Sweating is your body's normal response to a buildup of body heat. You sweat when you exercise or exert yourself, when you're in a warm environment, or when you're anxious or under stress. This type of sweating is both natural and healthy.

Sweating varies widely from person to person. Many women perspire more heavily during menopause. Drinking hot beverages, or beverages containing alcohol or caffeine, can trigger a light sweat for some individuals. Some people simply inherit a tendency to sweat heavily, especially on the soles of their feet and palms of their hands.

For most people, sweating, or perspiration, is a nuisance that feels uncomfortable and dampens clothing. Body odor is probably more troublesome. Although your sweat is practically odorless, it may take on an unpleasant or offensive odor when it comes into contact with bacteria on your skin.

Odor is more likely to develop at locations, such as your armpits and feet, that are more protected (for example, in shoes and socks) and tend to stay damp and warm. Sweating and body odor may also be influenced by your mood, your diet, some drugs and medical conditions, and even your hormone levels.

Because it's almost impossible to define what is a normal amount of sweating for everybody, try to learn what's normal for you. That may help you pinpoint any unusual changes.

A "cold sweat" is usually your body's response to serious illness, anxiety or severe pain. A cold sweat should receive immediate medical attention if there are signs of lightheadedness or chest and stomach pains.

Antiperspirants and deodorants

If you're concerned about sweating and body odor, the solution may be a simple one. Antiperspirants and deodorants can provide similar results, but they work in different ways:

- Antiperspirants contain aluminium-based compounds that temporarily block the sweat pore, thereby reducing the amount of perspiration that reaches your skin.
- Deodorants are usually alcohol-based and turn your skin acidic, making it less attractive to bacteria. Deodorants don't reduce perspiration but often contain fragrances to mask the odor.

The question of whether to choose an antiperspirant or deodorant depends on how much you sweat and how comfortable you are with that amount of sweat.

Medical help

Consult your doctor if you experience any of the following:

- You suddenly begin to sweat much more or less than usual.
- Sweating disrupts your daily routine.
- You experience night sweats for no apparent reason.
- You notice a change in body odor.

Excessive sweating associated with shortness of breath requires immediate medical attention. This could be a sign of a heart attack.

Home remedies

The following suggestions may help you reduce sweating and body odor:

- *Bathe daily.* Regular bathing helps keep the amount of bacteria on your skin in check.
- *Dry your feet thoroughly.* Microorganisms thrive in the damp spaces between your toes. Use over-the-counter foot powders to help absorb sweat.
- *Wear shoes made of natural materials.* Shoes made of materials such as leather or fabric help prevent sweaty feet by allowing your feet to breathe.
- *Rotate your shoes.* Shoes won't completely dry overnight, so try not to wear the same pair two days in a row if you have trouble with sweaty feet.
- *Wear the right socks.* Cotton and wool socks absorb moisture and help keep your feet dry. If you're active, moisture-wicking athletic socks are a good choice.
- *Change your socks often.* Change socks once or twice a day, drying your feet thoroughly each time. Women may prefer pantyhose with cotton soles.
- *Apply antiperspirants nightly.* At bedtime, apply antiperspirants to sweaty hands or feet. Try perfume-free antiperspirants.
- *Air your feet.* Go barefoot when you can, or at least slip out of your shoes now and then.
- *Choose natural-fiber clothing.* Wear fabrics such as cotton, wool and silk, which allow your skin to breathe. For exercise, you may prefer high-tech fabrics that can wick moisture away from your skin.
- *Try relaxation techniques.* Techniques such as yoga, meditation or biofeedback can help you control the stress that triggers perspiration.
- *Change your diet.* If certain foods or beverages cause you to sweat more than usual or your perspiration to smell, consider eliminating them from your diet.

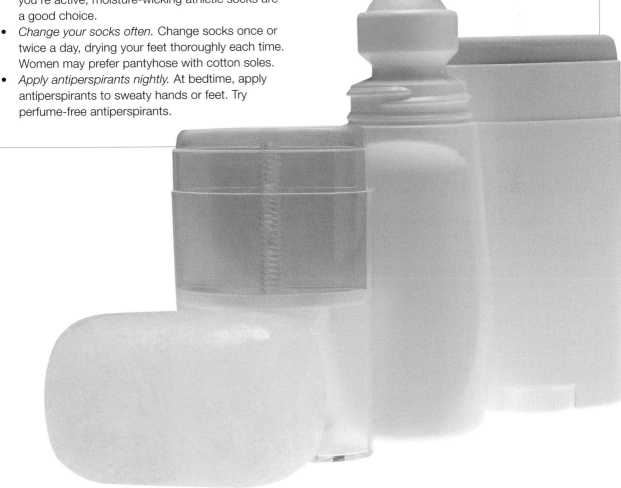

Swimmer's ear

Swimmer's ear, or otitis externa, is an infection of the ear canal. Your ear canal has features that help keep it clean and prevent infection, especially the substance you may know as earwax, or cerumen. Persistent moisture in the ear — for example, from frequent swimming — may result in a loss of earwax and breakdown of your defense against ear infection.

Swimmer's ear is most often caused by bacteria that are common in the environment. Infections caused by fungi or viruses are less common. Similar inflammation or infection may occur from scraping your ear canal while cleaning your ear or from hair sprays or hair dyes.

The signs and symptoms are generally mild at the onset, but may get worse if the infection isn't treated or it spreads. Signs and symptoms include:
- Redness in the ear canal
- Mild discomfort
- Drainage of clear fluid

These signs and symptoms may develop into ear pain, swelling, drainage of pus, and decreased or muffled hearing.

Medical help

See a doctor if you're experiencing any signs or symptoms of swimmer's ear, even if they are mild. Seek immediate medical care if you experience severe pain, significant drainage, fever or swelling, especially if you are immune suppressed or have diabetes.

Home remedies

If the discomfort is mild and there's no drainage from your ear, you can do the following:
- Place a warm (not hot) heating pad over your ear.
- Take aspirin or other over-the-counter pain medications (be sure to follow the label instructions).

Prevention

Follow these tips to prevent swimmer's ear:
- Keep your ears dry. Dry only your outer ear slowly and gently with a soft towel or cloth. Tip your head to the side to help water drain from your ear canal. Don't clean inside the ear canal unless you're instructed to do so by your doctor.
- Avoid getting water in your ear canal when bathing. Use a cotton ball coated with petroleum jelly to keep water out of your ears during showers and baths.
- Protect your ears. Avoid substances that may irritate your ears, such as hair sprays or hair dyes.
- Try a homemade preventive treatment. A mixture of 1 part white vinegar and 1 part rubbing alcohol may help prevent the growth of bacteria and fungi that can cause swimmer's ear. Apply before and after swimming. Pour 1 teaspoon of the solution into each ear and let it drain back out. Similar over-the-counter solutions may be available at your drugstore. You should not use vinegar and alcohol if you have a known hole (perforation) of the eardrum.

Swimmer's itch

Swimmer's itch is a rash caused by certain parasites that normally live on waterfowl and freshwater snails. On warm, sunny days — especially in calm freshwater lakes or ponds — these parasites can be released into the water.

During your swim, the parasites might burrow into your skin, where they cause an itchy rash. Fortunately, humans aren't suitable hosts for the parasites, which soon die.

Swimmer's itch is generally characterized by:

- Itching that may begin within an hour or two, or as long as two days, after swimming
- A red, raised rash

Swimmer's itch usually affects only exposed skin — skin not covered by swimsuits, wet suits or waders. Although uncomfortable, swimmer's itch is usually short-lived and typically clears on its own within a few days.

Medical help

Talk to your doctor if you have a rash after swimming that lasts more than one week. If you notice pus at the rash site, consult your doctor.

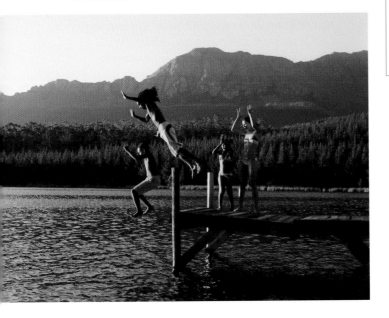

Home remedies

As much as you're tempted, don't scratch the affected areas. To relieve itching, try these remedies:

- Cover the rash with a clean, wet washcloth.
- Soak in a bath sprinkled with Epsom salts, baking soda or oatmeal.
- Stir water into baking soda until it makes a paste and then apply it to the affected areas.

Prevention

There's no evidence that applying sunscreen, lotions or creams helps prevent swimmer's itch. To reduce the risk of swimmer's itch:

- *Choose swimming spots carefully.* Avoid swimming in areas where swimmer's itch is a known problem or signs warn of possible contamination. Also avoid swimming or wading in marshy areas where snails are commonly found.
- *Avoid the shoreline, if possible.* If you're a strong swimmer, head to deeper water for your swim because you may be more likely to develop the itch if you spend a lot of time in shallow water.
- *Rinse after swimming.* Rinse exposed skin with fresh water immediately after the swim, then vigorously dry your skin with a towel. Launder your swimsuits often. You might even alternate between different swimsuits.
- *Take care of your pool.* If you have a pool, keep it well-maintained and chlorinated.

Teething

Teething occurs when a baby's teeth first begin to push through the gums. Although the timing varies widely, most babies begin teething by about age 6 months. The two bottom front teeth (lower central incisors) are usually the first to appear, followed by the two top front teeth (upper central incisors).

Classic signs and symptoms of teething include:

- Drooling, which may begin about two months before the first tooth appears
- Irritability or crankiness
- Swollen gums
- Chewing on solid objects

Many parents suspect that teething causes a fever and diarrhea, but researchers say this isn't true. Teething may cause signs and symptoms in the mouth and gums, but it doesn't cause problems elsewhere in the body.

Medical help

Teething can usually be handled at home. Contact the doctor if your baby develops a fever, seems particularly uncomfortable, or has other signs or symptoms of illness. The problem may be something other than teething.

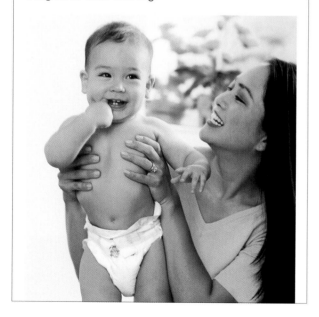

Home remedies

If your teething baby seems uncomfortable, consider these simple tips:

- *Rub your baby's gums.* Use a clean finger, moistened gauze pad or damp washcloth to massage your baby's gums. The pressure can ease your baby's discomfort.
- *Offer a teething ring.* Try one made of firm rubber. The liquid-filled variety may break under the pressure of your baby's chewing. If a bottle seems to do the trick, fill it with water. Prolonged contact with sugar from formula, milk or juice may cause tooth decay.
- *Keep it cool.* A cold washcloth or chilled teething ring can be soothing. Don't give your baby a frozen teething ring, however. Contact with extreme cold may hurt, doing your baby more harm than good. If your baby eats solid foods, offer items such as applesauce or yogurt.
- *Dry the drool.* Excessive drooling is part of the teething process. To prevent skin irritation, keep a clean cloth handy to dry your baby's chin. Have your baby sleep on an absorbent sheet.
- *Try an over-the-counter product.* If your baby is especially cranky, acetaminophen (Tylenol, others) or ibuprofen (Advil, Motrin IB, others) may help. Don't give your baby products that contain aspirin, however, and be cautious about teething medications that can be rubbed directly on a baby's gums. The medication may be washed away by your baby's saliva before it has any chance of doing good — and too much of the medication may numb your baby's throat, which may interfere with his or her normal gag reflex.

Tendinitis

Tendinitis is an inflammation or irritation of a tendon — one of the thick fibrous cords that attach muscles to bones. It can occur in any tendon, but is most common around your shoulders, elbows, wrists and heels. Common names for various tendinitis problems are tennis elbow, golfer's elbow, pitcher's shoulder, swimmer's shoulder and jumper's knee.

Signs and symptoms occur just outside the joint, at the point where a tendon attaches to a bone. They typically include:
- Pain, described as a dull ache
- Tenderness
- Mild swelling

Although tendinitis can be caused by injury from a sudden, single action, the condition is much more likely to stem from the repetition of a particular movement over time. Most people develop tendinitis because their jobs or their hobbies involve repetitive motions that aggravate the tendons needed to perform the tasks.

Tendinitis is also common in people whose daily activities involve awkward positions, frequent overhead reaching, vibration and forceful exertion.

Medical help

See your doctor if you have a fever, the area is inflamed or your symptoms don't improve within two weeks.

Home remedies

Although rest is a key part of treating tendinitis, prolonged inactivity can cause stiffness in your joints. After a few days of completely resting the injured area, gently move it through its full range of motion to maintain joint flexibility.
- Follow the instructions for P.R.I.C.E. (see page 157).
- Gently move the joint through its full range four times a day. Otherwise rest it. A sling, elastic bandage or splint may help.
- Take an anti-inflammatory medication such as aspirin, ibuprofen (Advil, Motrin IB, others), naproxen (Aleve) or products containing acetaminophen (Tylenol, others) to reduce the discomfort.

Prevention
To prevent tendinitis:
- *Ease up.* Avoid activities that place excessive stress on your tendons, especially for prolonged periods. If you notice pain, stop and rest.
- *Mix it up.* If one activity causes a persistent pain, try something else. Incorporate cross-training into your exercise program.
- *Improve your technique.* If your technique in an activity is flawed, you could be setting yourself up for tendon problems.
- *Stretch first.* Before you exercise, take time to stretch in order to maximize the range of motion in your joints.

Thumb pain

Pain at the base of your thumb may be the first sign of osteoarthritis in your hands, or you may be experiencing thumb arthritis or tendinitis of the thumb.

With any of these conditions, you may notice pain when you grip, grasp, pinch or apply force with your thumb. You may also experience swelling, and decreased strength and range of motion. It becomes difficult to perform simple tasks, such as writing, opening jars, turning the key in your door or car ignition, or trying to hold small objects.

With osteoarthritis of the hands, the pain may be limited to one joint or extend to many. It's more common in women than in men. Arthritis pain can be the result of a previous injury, repetitive activity or heredity. A common cause of thumb tendinitis is overuse of the wrist.

Medical help

If you have persistent swelling, stiffness or pain at the base of your thumb, you're unable to fully extend your thumb, or your thumb "catches" in a bent position, seek medical advice. Seek medical care immediately if the pain limits activities or is too severe to tolerate most days.

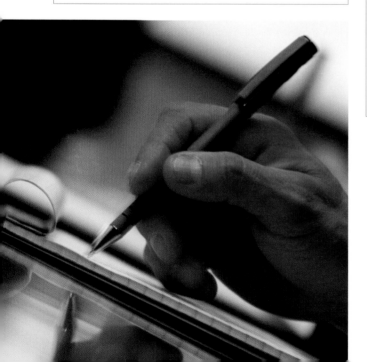

Home remedies

To help relieve thumb pain:
- *Take it easy.* Modify behaviors and avoid activities that cause pain.
- *Rest your thumb.* Use a splint to stabilize the wrist and thumb. Remove the splint at least four times a day to move and stretch the joints to maintain flexibility.
- *Use over-the-counter pain medications if the pain is severe.*
- *Apply heat or cold.* Alternate between heat and cold to help relieve swelling and pain and to soothe your joints. Heat can help ease pain, decrease joint stiffness and relax tense muscles. Experiment with hot packs or electric heating pads on their lowest settings, soaking your hands and wrists in warm water, or simply taking a warm shower or bath. Cold can be effective for reducing pain during flare-ups or after you've had too much physical activity. Applying ice packs or soaking your hands in cool or cold water has a numbing effect that dulls hand and wrist pain.
- *Exercise your thumb daily.* While your hands are warm, move your thumb in wide circles. Bend it to touch each of the other fingers on your hand.
- *Modify household equipment.* Consider purchasing adaptive equipment, such as jar openers, key turners and large zipper pulls. Enlarge the grasp on garden tools, kitchen utensils and writing devices — or buy items with large handles. Replace traditional door handles, which you must grasp with your thumb, with levers.

Tick bites

Spring and summer months are usually the time to worry about tick bites. Although the bites are often harmless, ticks can pass on organisms that may cause serious illnesses. Fortunately, antibiotic treatment is usually successful, particularly when treatment is started early.

Two of the most common tick-related diseases are Lyme disease and Rocky Mountain spotted fever. Although both illnesses can mimic other conditions, each may be identified by a telltale rash. Other tick-borne diseases include ehrlichiosis and anaplasmosis.

Lyme disease

Several days to weeks after a bite, a red, circular-shaped rash, often with a central clearing, may develop around the bite. Other indications may include:
- Flu-like signs and symptoms
- Pain that shifts from one joint to another
- Muscle aches

Rocky Mountain spotted fever

During the first week, a rash of red spots or blotches may appear on your wrists and ankles and eventually spread up your arms and legs to your chest. Other signs and symptoms include:
- High fever and chills
- Severe headache
- Abdominal pain
- Fatigue and loss of appetite

Medical help

Call your doctor if you can't completely remove the tick or you don't feel well. Also see your doctor if the tick was attached to your body for 36 hours or more, or you develop a rash, fever, stiff neck, muscle aches, joint pain and inflammation or flu-like symptoms.

Home remedies

To reduce your risk of getting a tick bite or becoming ill from the bite:
- When walking in wooded or grassy areas, wear shoes, long pants tucked into socks and light-colored, long-sleeved shirts. Avoid low bushes and long grass.
- Tick-proof your yard by clearing brush and leaves. Keep woodpiles in sunny areas.
- Check yourself and your pets often for ticks after being in wooded or grassy areas. Shower immediately after leaving these areas because ticks often remain on your skin for hours before biting.
- Insect repellents often repel ticks. Use products containing DEET or permethrin. Be sure to follow label precautions.

If you're bitten by a tick
- Remove the tick promptly and carefully. Use tweezers to grasp the tick near its head or mouth and pull gently and steadily to remove the whole tick without crushing it.
- If possible, seal the tick in a jar. Your doctor may want to see the tick if you develop signs and symptoms of illness after a tick bite.
- Use soap and water to wash your hands. Also wash the area around the tick bite after handling the tick.

Toenail fungal infections

Fungi are microscopic organisms that can invade your skin through tiny cuts or small separations between the nail and nail bed. Fungal infections occur more in toenails than in fingernails because toenails are often confined in a dark, warm moist environment inside your shoes — conditions perfect for the growth and spread of fungi.

This stubborn, but harmless, problem often begins as a tiny white or yellow spot on your toenail. Depending on the type of fungus, your nails may discolor, thicken, distort in shape or turn brittle, crumbly or ragged. The nail surface becomes dull, with no luster or shine.

Toenail fungal infections are more common among older adults. Other risk factors include perspiring heavily, working in a humid or moist environment, wearing footwear that inhibits good ventilation, having diabetes and having a damaged nail.

Medical help

If self-care measures aren't effective and the condition of your nails bothers you or causes problems, see your doctor or podiatrist.

Home remedies

To help prevent nail fungal infections, try the following steps:

- Avoid toenails that are too long or too short. Trim nails straight across and file down thickened areas.
- Keep your toenails dry and clean. Dry your feet thoroughly, including between your toes, after bathing.
- Change your socks often, especially if your feet sweat excessively. Take your shoes off occasionally during the day and after exercise. Synthetic socks that wick away moisture may keep your feet drier than do cotton or wool socks.
- Use antifungal spray or powder on your feet and inside your shoes.
- Don't trim or pick at the skin around your nails.
- Avoid walking barefoot in damp public places such as swimming pools, showers and locker rooms.

If a fungal infection is present, two home remedies that may be worth trying are:

- *Vinegar.* There's no evidence that a vinegar soak can cure nail fungus but some studies suggest that it may inhibit the growth of certain bacteria. Soak your feet for 15 to 20 minutes in a mixture of 1 part vinegar to 2 parts warm water. If your skin becomes irritated, try soaking only two to three times a week, or increase the proportion of water in the mixture.
- *Vicks VapoRub.* As with vinegar, there's no scientific proof that this product works on nail fungus, but anecdotal reports claim it does. You apply the product to infected nails but there's no consensus on how often.

Toothache

Tooth decay is the primary cause of toothaches. Bacteria that live in your mouth thrive on the sugars and starches in your food. These bacteria form a sticky plaque that clings to the surface of your teeth.

Decay-producing acid forms in plaque and attacks the hard outer coating (enamel) of your teeth. The erosion caused by plaque forms tiny openings (cavities) in tooth surfaces. The first sign of decay may be a sensation of pain when you eat something sweet, very cold or very hot. A tooth-ache often indicates that your dentist needs to check your teeth.

Tooth decay can occur more rapidly in people who have dry mouth, people who consume a lot of soft drinks or sports drinks or suck on hard candies or cough drops, people who eat a lot of high-sugar foods, and people who abuse methamphetamine.

Medical help

Contact your dentist if you have signs of infection, such as swelling, pain when you bite, red gums or a foul-tasting discharge. If a fever accompanies the pain, seek emergency care.

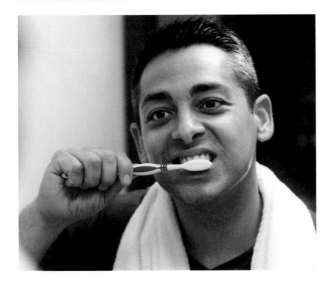

Home remedies

Until you're able to visit your dentist, try these self-care tips to help relieve toothache:

- Take an over-the-counter (OTC) pain reliever such as acetaminophen (Tylenol, others) and ibuprofen (Advil, Motrin IB, others).
- Apply an OTC gel containing benzocaine directly to the irritated tooth and gum. Direct application of oil of cloves (eugenol) also may help.
- Thoroughly clean all parts of your mouth, including all surfaces of your teeth — don't avoid the painful areas.
- Use warm water to brush your teeth.
- Use toothpaste designed for sensitive teeth.
- Avoid foods or beverages that are hot, cold or sweet enough to trigger pain.

Prevention

Taking good care of your teeth is the best way to avoid tooth decay and cavities.

- See your dentist twice a year.
- Brush your teeth at least twice a day — ideally after every meal — using a toothpaste that contains fluoride.
- Use floss or an interdental cleaner to remover food particles wedged between your teeth.
- If you can't brush after eating, try to rinse your mouth with mouthwash or water.
- Drink water that has fluoride added to it. The fluoride added to regular tap water has helped decrease tooth decay significantly. But today, many people drink bottled water that doesn't contain fluoride.

Traveler's diarrhea

Nothing can ruin a vacation or business trip faster than loose stools and abdominal cramps. Traveler's diarrhea usually isn't serious but it can be very disruptive and unpleasant.

A trip to a foreign country by no means guarantees gastrointestinal discomfort. But if you visit a place where the climate, social conditions or sanitary practices are different from yours at home, you have an increased risk of getting traveler's diarrhea.

It's possible that diarrhea while traveling may stem from the stress of travel or a change in diet. But a sudden change or high volume of output could be related to an infection from a virus, bacteria or parasite. You often get traveler's diarrhea from food or water contaminated by feces and organisms that you are not accustomed to.

The sickness strikes abruptly, usually lasts three to seven days and is rarely life-threatening. You generally don't require medical treatment other than replacing lost fluids, which can be made up with canned fruit juices, weak tea, clear soup and carbonated beverages.

Medical help

If you have severe dehydration, persistent vomiting, bloody stools or a high fever, or if your symptoms last for more than a few days, seek medical help. Be especially cautious with children, because traveler's diarrhea can cause severe dehydration in a short time.

Home remedies

Traveler's diarrhea tends to resolve itself but these medications may help relieve signs and symptoms:

- *Anti-motility agents.* These agents, including loperamide (Imodium) and medications containing diphenoxylate (Lomotil), provide prompt but temporary relief by slowing the transit time of food through your digestive tract and allowing more time for absorption.
- *Bismuth subsalicylate (Pepto Bismol).* This over-the-counter medication can decrease the frequency of your stools and shorten the duration of your illness. However, it isn't recommended for children, pregnant women or people who are allergic to aspirin.

Prevention

To reduce your risk of traveler's diarrhea:

- Avoid tap water or spring water. Drink only bottled water. Sodas, beer or wine served in their original containers are acceptable.
- Avoid ice cubes in your beverage. They may have been made with contaminated water.
- Use bottled water or boiled water to brush your teeth. Keep your mouth closed while showering.
- Don't eat any food from street vendors.
- Avoid salads, buffet foods, undercooked meats, raw vegetables, grapes, berries, fruits that have been peeled or cut, and unpasteurized milk and dairy products.
- Eat vegetables and fruits that you can peel yourself, such as bananas or oranges.

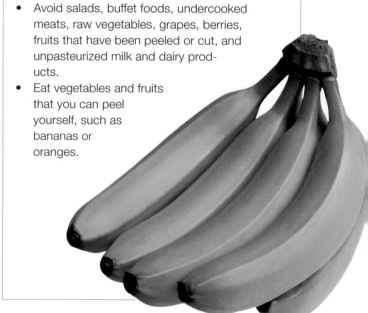

Ulcer

Peptic ulcers are open sores that develop on the inner lining of your esophagus, stomach or upper small intestine. It wasn't too long ago that lifestyle factors, such as a love of spicy foods or a stressful job, were thought to be at the root of most ulcers. Doctors now know that a *Helicobacter pylori* (*H. pylori*) bacterial infection — not stress or diet — is a primary cause of ulcers.

Burning pain is the most common symptom of an ulcer, and the pain is aggravated whenever stomach acid comes in direct contact with the ulcerated area. The pain typically may:

- Be felt anywhere from your navel up to your breastbone
- Last from a few minutes to several hours
- Be worse when your stomach is empty
- Flare at night
- Be relieved temporarily by eating certain foods or taking acid-reducing medication
- Disappear and then return for a few days or weeks

Medical help

An ulcer isn't something that you should treat on your own, without a doctor's help. Over-the-counter antacids and acid blockers may relieve the gnawing pain, but the relief is short-lived. If you have signs or symptoms of an ulcer, see your doctor for treatment.

Home remedies

To prevent ulcers or help existing ulcers heal, try the following:

- *Don't smoke.* Smoking may interfere with the protective function of your stomach lining, making it more susceptible to the development of an ulcer. Smoking also increases stomach acid.
- *Limit or avoid alcohol.* Excessive use of alcohol irritates and erodes the lining in your stomach and intestines, which can cause inflammation and bleeding.
- *Avoid nonsteroidal anti-inflammatory drugs (NSAIDs).* These products can irritate your stomach lining. Seek medical advice if you must use pain relievers regularly
- *Control acid reflux.* If you have an esophageal ulcer — usually associated with acid reflux — you can take steps to help manage the reflux. These include avoiding spicy or fatty foods, avoiding lying down after meals, reducing your weight and raising the head of your bed.
- *Avoid trigger foods.* While an ulcer is healing, it's advisable to watch what you eat. Acidic or spicy foods may increase stomach acid, increasing ulcer pain. So can beverages that contain caffeine.
- *Control stress while healing.* If stress is severe, it may delay the healing of an ulcer.

Vaginal yeast infection

A vaginal yeast infection is a type of vaginitis — inflammation of the vagina — typically caused when the balance of microorganisms that are normally present in your vagina becomes altered. These changes may result in an overgrowth of yeast, which can lead to a yeast infection. The signs and symptoms of infection can range from mild to severe, including:

- Itching and irritation in the vagina and at the entrance to the vagina (vulva)
- Burning sensation, especially during intercourse or while urinating
- Red, swollen vulva
- Vaginal pain and soreness
- Thick, white, odor-free vaginal discharge with a cottage cheese appearance

You're more susceptible to a yeast infection if you are pregnant or have diabetes, or if you're taking antibiotics, cortisone or birth control pills.

Medical help

Make an appointment to see your doctor if:
- This is the first time you've experienced a yeast infection
- You're not sure whether you have a yeast infection
- Your symptoms don't go away after self-treating with anti-fungal creams and suppositories
- You develop other symptoms

Home remedies

Treatment options include one-day, three-day and seven-day courses of medications for yeast infections. The active ingredient in these creams or suppositories is clotrimazole (Gyne-Lotrimin), miconazole (Monistat) or tioconazole (Vagistat). Some of these products also come with an external cream that is applied to the labia and vulva to soothe itching. Follow package directions and complete the entire course of treatment, even if you're feeling better right away.

To ease discomfort until an antifungal medication takes full effect, apply a cold compress, such as a damp washcloth, to the labial area. You may also take probiotic supplements or suppositories. Probiotics contain beneficial bacteria, such as *Lactobacillus acidophilus*, which may help restore the balance of microorganisms in your vagina. One study found that suppositories containing *L. acidophilus* improved symptoms of vaginal yeast infections, while other studies of oral preparations of *L. acidophilus* found little benefit. Eating yogurt that contains active lactobacillus cultures is a healthy habit, but more research is needed to determine whether it is helpful for yeast infections.

Prevention
To help prevent vaginal yeast infections, try the following:
- *Don't douche.* The vagina doesn't require cleansing other than normal bathing. Repetitive douching disrupts the balance of organisms that normally live in the vagina. And douching won't clear up an infection of the vagina.
- *Avoid potential irritants, such as scented tampons or pads.*
- *Wear cotton underwear and pantyhose with a cotton crotch.* Don't wear underwear to bed. Yeast thrives in moist environments.
- *Change out of wet swimsuits and damp clothing as soon as possible.*

Varicose veins

Varicose veins are gnarled, enlarged veins that you can see just under the surface of your skin. They may be blue or dark purple in color. Any vein may become varicose, but the veins most commonly affected are those in your legs and feet.

For many people, varicose veins don't cause any pain and are primarily a cosmetic concern. But for some people, they cause aching pain and discomfort or chronic leg wounds. Sometimes varicose veins signal a higher risk of other circulatory problems.

If painful signs and symptoms do occur, they may include:

- Achy feeling in your legs
- Burning, throbbing, muscle cramping and swelling in your lower legs
- Worsened pain after sitting or standing for a long time
- Itching around one or more of your veins
- Skin ulcers near your ankle or lower legs, which may signal vein concerns that require medical attention.

Medical help

If you're concerned about how your veins look and feel and self-care measures haven't helped, consult your doctor. See your doctor if you develop skin ulcers or if the veins become sore or reddened and one leg is more swollen than the other.

Home remedies

These steps may decrease the discomfort of varicose veins and help prevent or slow their development, as well. They include:

- *Exercise.* Get your legs moving. Walking is a great way to encourage blood circulation in your legs.
- *Watch your weight and your diet.* Shedding excess pounds takes pressure off your veins. Follow a low-salt, high-fiber diet to prevent the swelling that may result from water retention and constipation.
- *Watch what you wear.* Avoid high heels. Low-heeled shoes work calf muscles more, which is better for your veins. Don't wear tight clothes around your waist, legs or groin. Tight underwear or hosiery, for instance, can cut off blood flow.
- *Elevate your legs.* To improve circulation in your legs, take short breaks daily to elevate your legs above the level of your heart. For example, lie down with your legs resting on three or four pillows.
- *Avoid long periods of sitting or standing.* Make a point of changing your position frequently to encourage blood flow. Try to move around at least every 30 minutes. If able, consider a standing or treadmill workstation.
- *Don't sit with your legs crossed.* Some doctors believe this position can increase the risk of circulation problems.
- *Wear compression socks when traveling or standing for long periods of time.* A compression level of at least 10 to 20 millimeters of mercury (mm Hg) is best.

Warts

Common warts are caused by a virus that triggers a rapid growth of cells on the outer layer of your skin. The warts look like small, grainy bumps that are rough to the touch. They may be painful and unsightly, but they're usually harmless and often disappear on their own without treatment. Common warts aren't cancerous.

There are more than 200 types of warts. Common warts usually occur on your hands and fingers. Other types of warts include:

- Plantar warts, which occur on the soles of your feet
- Genital warts, which develop in your genital area
- Flat warts, which often appear on your face, hands and legs

Like other infectious diseases, wart viruses pass from person to person. It can take a wart as long as two to six months to develop after your skin has been exposed to the virus.

Medical help

Most warts disappear on their own or with self-care. Prompt treatment by a doctor, however, may decrease the chance that the warts will spread. Also visit your doctor if your warts are a cosmetic nuisance, bothersome, painful or rapidly multiplying.

Home remedies

Unless you have an impaired immune system or diabetes, try these home remedies to remove warts:

Salicylic acid

Wart-removal products are available at drugstores, either as a topical solution or patch. For common warts, look for products containing 17 percent salicylic acid (Compound W, Occlusal-HP), which peels off the infected skin. These products require daily use, often for a few weeks. For best results, soak your wart in warm water for 10 to 20 minutes before applying the product. File away any dead skin with a nail file or pumice stone between treatments. Just be careful — the acid in these products can irritate or damage healthy skin around the wart. If you're pregnant, talk with your doctor before using an acid solution.

Freezing

Some liquid nitrogen products are available in nonprescription liquid or spray form.

Duct tape

One study employed a "duct tape therapy" that involved covering warts with duct tape for six days, then soaking the warts in warm water and rubbing them with an emery board or pumice stone. The process was repeated for as long as two months. Researchers hypothesized that this unconventional therapy worked by irritating the wart and triggering the body's immune system to attack the virus. Further study results have been mixed on the effectiveness of duct tape in removing warts, either alone or with other therapies.

Watery eyes

Tears lubricate your eyes and help wash away particles of dust and grit. Watery eyes occur when an excess production of tears overwhelms your eyelids or when the fluid drains too slowly through your tear ducts.

One of the most common causes of watery eyes is an age-related change affecting your eyelids. As you get older, the muscles in your eyelids tend to relax, which may prevent the inner lid from lying flat against the eye's surface. The result is a pooling of tears in the corners of your eyes. The tears remain and may become stagnant, irritating your eyes.

Another common age-related cause of tearing is when a tear duct becomes blocked, preventing the drainage of fluid from the eye. Other causes include dryness and irritation from the environment. Watery eyes commonly accompany infections such as pink eye. They can also result from allergies, including an allergic reaction to preservatives in eyedrops or contact lens solutions.

Medical help

Seek medical care if the condition continues despite self-care efforts and interferes with your daily activities, or if you develop eye pain or a new onset of impaired vision.

Home remedies

To help treat and prevent watery eyes:
- Apply a warm compress over closed eyelids two to four times a day for 10 minutes.
- Don't rub your eyes.
- Replace mascara and other types of eye makeup at least every three months. These products can become contaminated with bacteria transferred by the applicator.
- Follow proper directions for the wearing, cleaning and disinfecting of contact lenses.

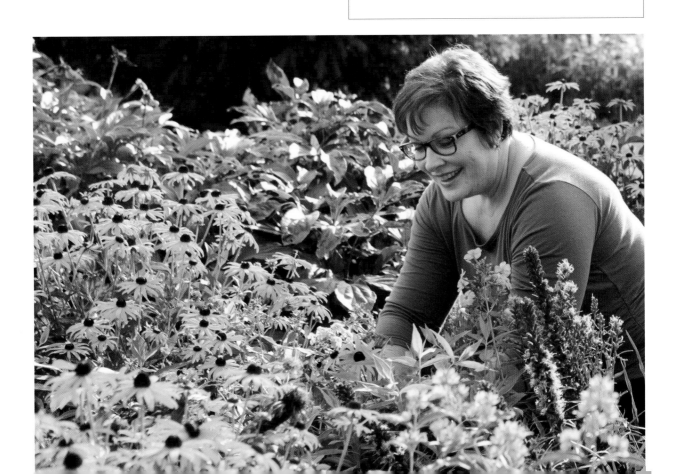

Wrinkles

Wrinkles are a natural part of aging. As you grow older, your skin gets thinner, drier, less elastic and less able to protect itself from damage. As a result, wrinkles, lines and creases form on your skin.

Some people don't seem to age as quickly as others do. Although genetics is the most important factor in determining skin texture, another major contributor to wrinkles is spending too much time in the sun. Smoking also can cause premature aging of your skin.

Cosmetic products that promise youthful skin are often expensive and usually fail to deliver any significant improvements. When wrinkles become bothersome, people often turn to medications, resurfacing techniques, fillers, injectables and surgery to help smooth and invigorate their skin.

Medical help

If you're concerned about the appearance of your skin, see your dermatologist. He or she can help you create a personalized skin-care plan by assessing your skin type and evaluating your skin's condition. A dermatologist can also recommend medical wrinkle treatments.

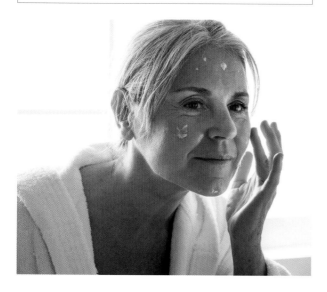

Home remedies

These measures may help slow the process of aging skin:

- *Protect your skin from the sun.* Shield your skin — and help prevent future wrinkles — by limiting the amount of time you spend in the sun. Always wear protective clothing and hats outdoors. Also, use sunscreen when outdoors, even in winter.
- *Choose products with built-in sunscreen.* When selecting skin-care products, choose those with a built-in sun protection factor (SPF) of at least 15. Also, be sure to select products that block both types of ultraviolet (UVA and UVB) rays.
- *Use moisturizers.* Dryness turns plump skin cells into shriveled ones, creating fine lines and wrinkles long before you're due. Though moisturizers can't prevent wrinkles, they may temporarily mask tiny lines and creases. Also avoid harsh soaps and hot water when bathing.
- *Don't smoke.* Even if you've smoked for years or smoked heavily when you were younger, you can still improve your skin tone and texture and prevent future wrinkles by quitting smoking.

Not all wrinkle creams are equal

The effectiveness of anti-wrinkle creams depends in part on the active ingredient or ingredients they contain. Retinol, alpha hydroxy acid, kinetin, coenzyme Q10, copper peptides and antioxidants may result in slight to modest improvements in wrinkles. However, wrinkle creams containing these ingredients that are sold over-the-counter contain lower concentrations of these active ingredients than do prescription creams. Therefore, the results — if any — are limited and usually short-lived.

Wrist and hand pain

Think of all the things you do each day using your wrists, hands and fingers. You may not even be aware of the many nerves, blood vessels, muscles and small bones that work together as you perform a task as simple as turning a key in the door — until the movement becomes painful.

Pain may be caused by sudden injuries such as sprains or fractures. But long-term medical problems also may cause wrist and hand pain, such as arthritis, carpal tunnel syndrome and the wear and tear from overuse or repetitive movements.

The amount of pain may vary, depending on what's causing it. For example, pain from osteoarthritis is often described as similar to a dull toothache, while tendinitis usually causes a sharp, stabbing pain. The location of pain also may provide clues as to what is causing signs and symptoms.

Ganglion cysts

Ganglion cysts are fluid-filled lumps that usually appear along tendons and joints of your wrists and hands. Ganglions are sometimes painful and, if bothersome, may require treatment. Seek medical care immediately if a lump becomes painful and inflamed or if a cyst breaks through the skin and begins to drain.

Home remedies

To relieve wrist and hand pain:
- Follow the instructions for P. R.I.C.E. (see page 157).
- Use over-the-counter pain medications, if needed.

Prevention

To prevent wrist and hand problems:
- Build bone strength with a diet that includes adequate amounts of calcium and vitamin D to prevent fractures.
- Use tools with large handles so you don't have to grip them as hard.
- Remove rings from your fingers before doing manual labor. If you injure your hand, remove rings before your fingers become swollen.
- Take frequent breaks to rest muscles you're using regularly, and try to vary activities so you're not always using the same muscles.
- Do flexibility and strengthening exercises.
- Try out special ergonomic devices that can make you more comfortable, improve posture and protect your wrists and hands.

Medical help

Minor sprains and strains usually respond to rest, ice and over-the-counter pain medications. But if pain and swelling last longer than a few days or becomes worse, see your doctor. Seek medical care immediately if:
- You suspect a fracture
- A fall or accident has caused rapid swelling and moving the area is painful
- The area is hot and inflamed and you have a fever

Emergency care

Emergencies don't happen every day, but when they do, there is usually little time to react, and help may not be immediately at hand. With preparation, you can respond effectively when a person appears injured, seriously ill or in distress. Perhaps this preparation may never be needed, but on the chance it is, your quick action could someday save a life.

Take a certified first-aid training course to learn lifesaving skills, such as cardiopulmonary resuscitation (CPR) and the Heimlich maneuver, and to recognize signs of heart attack, shock and traumatic injury. Check with your local American Red Cross, county emergency services, public safety office or the American Heart Association for information on first aid and related courses that are offered in your community.

In this section, we discuss some of the basic steps you may take in case of an emergency until medical help arrives.

Allergic reaction (anaphylaxis)

Anaphylaxis is a severe, potentially life-threatening allergic reaction. It can occur rapidly after you're exposed to something that you're allergic to, such as peanuts or venom from a bee sting.

Normally, your immune system functions by producing chemicals that help protect you from foreign substances, including bacteria and viruses. Infrequently, however, your system overreacts. During anaphylaxis, your immune system releases a flood of chemicals that puts your entire body into shock. Your blood pressure drops suddenly and your airways constrict, preventing you from breathing normally.

Anaphylaxis requires an immediate trip to the emergency room and an injection of epinephrine to reduce your body's allergic response. If your condition isn't treated quickly, it can lead to unconsciousness or death.

Signs and symptoms

An anaphylactic reaction is most likely to occur soon after exposure to the allergy trigger (allergen). Even if, in the past, you only experienced a mild reaction to a particular allergen, you still may be at risk of a severe reaction when you're exposed to it again.

Signs and symptoms of a reaction usually occur within seconds or minutes of exposure to the allergen. In some cases, the reaction occurs more than a half-hour after the exposure.

Anaphylactic signs and symptoms include:
- Skin reactions, such as hives, swollen eyes, itching and skin that is flushed, pale or cool and clammy
- Constricted airways and swollen lips, tongue or throat, which can cause wheezing and trouble breathing
- Weak and rapid pulse
- Nausea, vomiting or diarrhea
- Dizziness or fainting

Triggers

A number of allergens can trigger anaphylaxis, depending on how sensitive you are to different substances. Some common triggers include:
- Foods such as peanuts, tree nuts (walnuts, pecans), fish, shellfish, milk and eggs
- Insect stings from bees, yellow jackets, wasps, hornets and fire ants
- Certain medications, especially penicillin

What to do

If someone is having a severe allergic reaction and showing signs of shock, quick action is essential. Even if you're not positive of the cause, take the following steps immediately:
- Call 911 or emergency medical help.
- Check the person's pulse and breathing and, if necessary, use CPR or other first aid.
- If the person has medications to treat an allergy attack, such as an epinephrine auto-injector, give it immediately.

Using an autoinjector

Many people at risk of anaphylaxis carry a device called an autoinjector. This device is a spring-loaded syringe that can inject a single dose of medication when pressed against the thigh. The device is generally very easy to use and instructions are often printed on the side.

If you require an autoinjector, make sure that you, as well as the people closest to you, know how to administer the drug. If family or friends are with you in an anaphylactic emergency, they could save your life. Medical personnel responding to a call for help also may give you an injection of epinephrine or another medication to treat your symptoms.

Bleeding

Bleeding may occur externally through cuts and tears in the skin or internally from ruptured blood vessels, sometimes exiting through natural openings of the body such as the mouth. Most injuries don't cause life-threatening bleeding, but in situations where substantial blood is lost, shock, unconsciousness and death may result.

To stop severe bleeding, follow these steps:

1. Lay a bleeding person down and, if possible, cover his or her body with a blanket or jacket to prevent the loss of heat.
2. If possible, position the person's head slightly lower than his or her trunk or elevate the legs. This position reduces the risk of fainting by increasing blood flow to the brain. If possible, elevate the site that's bleeding.
3. While wearing gloves, remove any obvious dirt or debris from the wound. Don't remove objects that are embedded in the skin. Don't probe into the wound or attempt to clean or rinse it out. Your primary concern is to stop the bleeding.
4. Apply direct pressure on the wound, using a sterile bandage, clean cloth, article of clothing or, if nothing else, your hands.
5. Hold continuous pressure on the wound for at least 20 minutes without checking to see if the bleeding has stopped. Then, maintain pressure by binding the wound with a bandage or clean cloth and adhesive tape. Don't apply a tourniquet except as a last resort.
6. Don't remove the gauze or bandage. If bleeding continues and begins to seep through the material you're holding on the wound, add more absorbent layers of material on top of it.
7. If direct pressure on the wound doesn't stop the bleeding, you can apply pressure to the main artery that delivers blood to the area of the wound. Squeeze the artery against nearby bone while keeping your fingers flat. With the other hand, continue to apply pressure on the wound.
8. Immobilize the body part that's injured — in other words, try to keep it in a stable position — once the bleeding has been stopped. Leave the bandages in place and call 911 or your emergency medical help. Transport the injured person to an emergency room as soon as possible if there is severe bleeding or signs of shock.

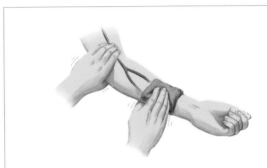

To stop bleeding, apply pressure directly to the wound using a sterile bandage, gauze or clean cloth.

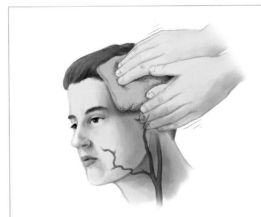

If bleeding continues despite pressure applied directly to the wound, maintain pressure and also apply pressure to the nearest major artery between the injury and the heart.

Burns

The most serious burns — third-degree burns — are an emergency involving all layers of skin and causing permanent tissue damage (see page 33). The burned areas may be charred black or appear dry and white. If smoke inhalation accompanies the burn, breathing may be difficult. You may have carbon monoxide poisoning or other toxic effects.

For severe burns

Call 911 or emergency medical help. Until an emergency unit arrives, follow these steps:

- Don't try to remove burned clothing. However, do make sure the victim is not in contact with smoldering materials or exposed to smoke or heat.
- Don't immerse large burns in cold water or ice. Doing so could cause a drop in body temperature and reduce blood pressure and circulation, putting the body in shock.
- Elevate the body part or parts that are burned. Raise them above heart level, if possible.
- Gently cover the burned area. Use a cool, moist, sterile bandage, cloth or towel.

For electrical burns

An electrical burn may appear minor or not show on a person's skin, but the damage can extend deep into underlying tissues below the surface. If a strong electrical current passes through the body, internal damage, such as a heart rhythm disturbance or cardiac arrest, can occur.

Sometimes the jolt associated with an electrical burn can throw a person to the ground or against a wall, resulting in fractures or other injuries.

Call 911 or emergency medical help if the person who has been burned is in pain, is confused, or is experiencing any changes in breathing, pulse or consciousness.

While waiting for medical help to arrive, follow these steps:

1. Don't touch. The person may still be in contact with the electrical source. Touching the person may pass the current through you.
2. Turn off the power source, if possible. If you're unable to do so, try to move the source away from both you and the injured person using a dry, nonconducting object made of cardboard, plastic or wood. Don't attempt this if the voltage is over 600 volts, such as a downed power line.
3. Check for breathing and pulse. If absent, begin CPR on the individual immediately.

For chemical burns

Make sure the cause of the burn has been removed. Flush chemicals off the skin's surface with cool running water for at least 10 minutes. If the burning chemical is a powderlike substance such as lime, brush it off your skin before flushing.

Remove clothing and jewelry that has been contaminated by the chemical. Then, wrap the area with a dry, sterile dressing (if possible) or clean cloth.

Seek emergency assistance if:

- The person shows signs of shock, such as fainting, pale complexion or breathing in a notably shallow manner
- The chemical burn has penetrated through the upper skin layer, and the burned area exceeds 3 inches in diameter
- The chemical burn occurred on an eye, face, hand, foot, groin or buttock, or over a major joint

If you need to seek medical care, bring the container if possible so that medical personnel know the type of chemical causing the burn.

Cardiopulmonary resuscitation (CPR)

Cardiopulmonary resuscitation (CPR) can save lives in a range of emergencies, such as a heart attack or near drowning, in which someone's breathing or heartbeat has stopped.

Ideally, CPR involves two separate elements: chest compressions combined with mouth-to-mouth rescue breathing. But what you are able to perform in an emergency situation depends on your knowledge and comfort level. If you're untrained or unsure of your skills, you may do "hands-only" CPR (chest compressions) and not mouth-to-mouth rescue breathing (see more on page 399).

The bottom line is: It's far better to do something than to do nothing at all — the difference could save a person's life.

Before you begin

Before starting CPR, check:
- Is the environment safe for the person?
- Is the person conscious or unconscious?
- If the person is unresponsive and appears to be unconscious, tap or shake the shoulder and ask loudly, "Are you OK?"

- If there's no response, and another person is able to help you, one of you should call 911 or emergency medical help while the other begins CPR. If you're alone but have immediate access to a telephone, call the emergency number before starting CPR.
- If an automated external defibrillator (AED) is immediately available, bring it near the unconscious person. Voice prompts from the device will guide you step by step on its use (see box below for more). If advised to do so by the voice prompts, deliver one shock, and then begin CPR.

CPR

When performing CPR, your actions should be performed in a specific sequence that's best described as the CAB method — which stands for compressions, airway and breathing.

C. Compressions to restore circulation
After you've delivered one shock from an AED, or if an AED is unavailable, begin CPR by starting chest compressions:

How AEDs work

An automated external defibrillator (AED) is a device that senses your heart's rhythm during cardiac arrest and, in some cases, delivers an electric shock to get your heart beating again.

A short instructional video typically accompanies the AED that explains how to use and maintain the device. Watch the video after your purchase, and periodically review how to use it later on.

In an emergency, the AED will essentially make decisions for you. Voice instructions guide you through the defibrillation process, explaining how to check for breathing and pulse, and how to position electrode pads on the person's chest.

Once the pads are in place, the AED automatically measures the heart rhythms. If a shock is needed, the device will instruct you on delivering it. The AED will also guide you through CPR. The process can be repeated as needed until emergency responders take over.

CPR (continued)

1. Put the person on his or her back on a firm surface.
2. Kneel next to the person's neck and shoulders.
3. Place the heel of one hand over the center of the person's chest, between the nipples. Place your other hand on top of the first hand. Keep your elbows straight and position your shoulders directly above your hands.
4. Use your upper body weight (not just your arms) as you push straight down on (compress) the chest 2 to 2.4 inches. Push hard at a rate of 100 to 120 compressions a minute.
5. If you haven't been trained in CPR, continue chest compressions until there are signs of movement or until emergency medical personnel take over. If you have been trained in CPR, go on to checking the airway and rescue breathing.

A. Clear the airway

1. If you're trained in CPR and you've performed 30 chest compressions, open the person's airway using the head-tilt, chin-lift maneuver. Put your palm on the person's forehead and gently tilt the head back. Then with the other hand, gently lift the chin forward to open the airway.
2. Check for normal breathing, taking no more than five or 10 seconds. Look for chest motion, listen for normal breath sounds, and feel for the person's breath on your cheek and ear. Gasping is not considered to be normal breathing. If the person isn't breathing normally and you are trained in CPR, begin mouth-to-mouth breathing. If you believe the person is unconscious from a heart attack and you haven't been trained in emergency procedures, skip mouth-to-mouth breathing and continue chest compressions.

B. Breathe for the person

Rescue breathing can be mouth-to-mouth or mouth-to-nose if the mouth is seriously injured or can't be opened.

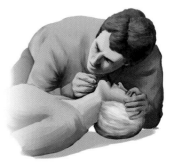

Use your upper body weight as you push straight down (compress) the chest about 2 inches.

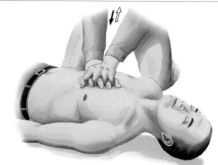

Take no more than 10 seconds to check for normal breathing. Look for chest motion, listen for breath sounds, and feel for breath on your cheek and ear.

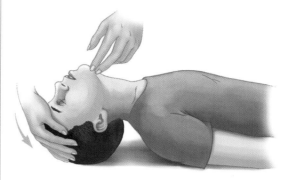

Put your palm on the forehead and gently tilt the head back. With your other hand, gently lift the chin forward to open the airway.

CPR

1. With the airway open (head tilted, chin lifted) pinch the nostrils shut and cover the person's mouth with yours, making a seal.
2. Prepare to give two breaths. Give the first breath, lasting one second. If the chest rises, give the second breath. If the chest doesn't rise, repeat the head-tilt, chin-lift maneuver, and then give the second breath. Thirty chest compressions followed by two rescue breaths is considered one cycle. Be careful not to provide too many breaths or to breathe with too much force.
3. Resume chest compressions to restore circulation at the same rate as before.
4. If the person has not begun moving after five cycles (about two minutes) and an automated

external defibrillator (AED) is available, apply it and follow the prompts. Administer one shock, and then resume CPR — starting with chest compressions — for two more minutes before administering a second shock. If you're not trained to use an AED, a 911 or other emergency medical operator may be able to guide you in its use. If an AED isn't available, go to step 5 below.
5. Continue CPR until there are signs of movement or until emergency medical responders can take over.

CPR for children

For children ages 1 to puberty, perform CPR first, and then call 911 or emergency medical help. If you're alone with an infant or a child, perform five cycles (two minutes) of CPR before calling for help or using an AED. Use one or two hands (depending on the child's size) and breathe more gently.

CPR for infants

The procedure for giving CPR to an infant (under 12 months old) is similar to the one used for adults. Loudly call out the infant's name and

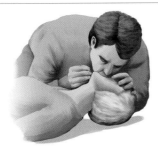

With the airway open, pinch the nostrils shut and cover the person's mouth with yours. Give the breath.

Hands-only CPR saves lives

The American Heart Association (AHA) states that bystanders can effectively use hands-only CPR — chest compressions without rescue breaths — on adults or adolescents in emergency situations if the bystanders have witnessed the event. Hands-only CPR involves:
1. Calling 911 or emergency medical help
2. Giving chest compressions, pushing hard and fast in the center of the chest and avoiding interruptions. The compressions continue until emergency medical responders arrive and say to stop.
   Bystanders should also try to perform traditional CPR (with rescue breaths) if they don't witness the event.

CPR (continued)

stroke or gently tap the shoulder. Do not shake the child. If there's no response, have someone call 911 or emergency medical help while you follow:

Compression

1. Place the infant on his or her back on a firm, flat surface, such as a table or the floor.
2. Image a horizontal line drawn between the baby's nipples. Place two fingers of one hand just below this line, in the center of the chest.
3. Gently compress the chest about 1.5 inches. Count aloud as you push in fairly rapid rhythm (a rate of about 100 compressions a minute).

Airway

1. After 30 compressions, gently tip the head back by lifting the chin with one hand and pushing down on the forehead with the other hand.
2. In no more than 10 seconds, check for signs of breathing: Look for chest motion, listen for breath sounds, and feel for breath on your cheek and ear.

Breathing

1. Cover the mouth and nose with your mouth.
2. Prepare to give two gentle breaths. Use the strength of your cheeks to deliver puffs of air instead of deep breaths from your lungs.
3. After the first breath, watch to see if the chest rises. If it does, give a second breath. If it doesn't, repeat the head-tilt, chin-lift maneuver and give the second breath.
4. If the baby's chest still doesn't rise, examine the mouth to make sure no foreign material is inside. If an object is seen, sweep it out with your finger. If the airway seems blocked perform first aid for a choking baby (see page 402).

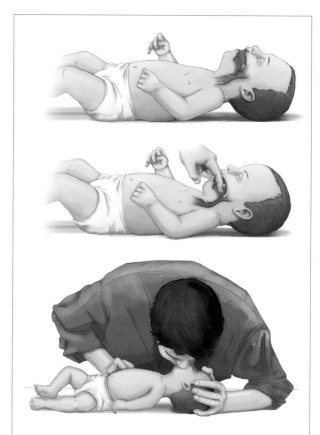

Tilt the child's head back to open the airway. If you see an object in the infant's mouth, remove it with a sweep of your finger. Alternate compression of the infant's chest with gentle breaths from your mouth.

5. Give two rescue breaths after every 30 chest compressions. If someone else can help you provide CPR, one person does 15 chest compressions and the other person delivers the two rescue breaths.
6. Perform CPR for two minutes before making an emergency call for help, unless someone else can make the call while you attend to the infant.
7. Continue CPR until you see signs of life or until emergency responders arrive.

Choking

Choking occurs when an object becomes lodged in your throat or windpipe, stopping the flow of air to your lungs. The blockage, in turn, cuts off the circulation of oxygen-rich blood to your brain and other vital organs. If the blockage isn't cleared rapidly, the condition can prove fatal.

A common cause of blockage is food — often from eating too fast or while laughing, talking or doing some form of physical activity.

The universal sign of choking is hands clutched to the throat. If a person in distress doesn't give this indication, look for other signs:

- Inability to talk
- Difficulty breathing or noisy breathing
- Inability to cough forcefully
- Skin, lips and nails turning blue or dusky
- Loss of consciousness

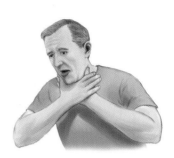

Typically, a person who is choking is unable to communicate except by hand motions.

Five-and-five approach

For situations in which a person is choking, the Red Cross recommends that you take a "five-and-five" approach:

1. Give five blows to the back between the shoulder blades using the heel of your hand.
2. Deliver five abdominal thrusts. These thrusts are known as the Heimlich maneuver.
3. Continue to alternate between five back blows and five abdominal thrusts until the blockage is dislodged.

If you're alone, do the five-and-five approach before calling 911 or emergency medical help. If another person is present, have that person call for help while you give first aid. If the person becomes unconscious during the procedure, perform CPR with chest compressions (see pages 189-191).

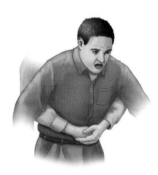

The Heimlich maneuver should be performed if the person can't speak, cough or effectively breathe.

The Heimlich maneuver

The Heimlich maneuver is perhaps the best known technique for clearing an obstructed airway. It should be used on someone only if there's a complete or near-complete blockage of the airway. To perform the maneuver:

1. Stand behind the person. Wrap your arms around the person's waist. Tip the person forward slightly.
2. Make a fist with one hand. Place it slightly above the person's navel.
3. Grasp the fist with your other hand. Press hard into the abdomen with a quick, upward thrust, as if trying to lift the person up.
4. Continue the five-and-five cycle until the blockage is dislodged.

Choking (continued)

When a child is choking

If the child is older than 1 year, use the Heimlich maneuver. If the child is under 1 year, sit down and hold the child face down on your forearm, which should be resting on your thigh. The infant's head is slightly lower than the chest.

Gently but firmly thump between the shoulder blades with the heel of your hand five times. The combination of gravity and force should release the object that's blocking the airway.

If the blockage isn't released, hold the infant on your forearm, face up with the head lower than the trunk. Place two fingers on the breastbone and give five quick chest compressions.

Repeat the back thumps and chest compressions if breathing doesn't resume. Call for emergency help. If you open the airway but there's no breathing, begin CPR for infants (see pages 191-192).

When a person is unconscious

1. Lower the person on his or her back to the floor, if he or she isn't already lying down.
2. Try to clear the airway. If there is visible blockage in the throat, reach a finger into the mouth and sweep out the cause of the blockage. Be careful not to push the object deeper into the airway.
3. Begin CPR if the object remains lodged and the person doesn't respond to the above measures. Chest compressions used in CPR could help to dislodge the object. Remember to recheck the mouth periodically.

When you're alone

If you're alone and choking, back blows aren't an option. However, you can perform abdominal thrusts to dislodge the blockage.

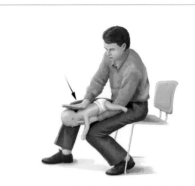

A gentle thump on the back can help clear the airway of a choking infant.

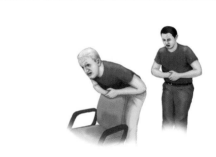

If help is unavailable, you can perform the Heimlich maneuver on yourself.

1. Make a fist and place it above your navel, with the thumb side toward your abdomen.
2. Grasp your fist with the other hand and bend over a hard surface — a chair or countertop will do.
3. Shove your fist inward and upward. Continue to do so until the object dislodges.

Fracture

A bone fracture usually occurs as a result of a fall, blow or other traumatic event. If you suspect a fracture, protect the injury from further damage. Don't try to realign the injured bone. Instead, try to immobilize it in a stable position — including any joint above and below the injury. A firm pillow or other firm item may help you.

A fracture requires medical attention. If a broken bone is the result of major trauma, call 911 or emergency medical help.

Signs and symptoms

Signs and symptoms of a fracture may include:
- Swelling or bruising over a bone
- Limb deformity
- Sharp pain that intensifies when the affected area is moved or pressure is put on it
- Loss of function in injured area
- Broken bone that has poked through the skin

If bleeding occurs with the broken bone, apply pressure to stop the bleeding. If possible, elevate the wound to lessen blood flow. Maintain pressure on the wound for at least 15 minutes. If bleeding continues, reapply pressure until it stops.

If you've been trained in the procedure and professional help isn't available, you may use a simple splint to immobilize a fractured area. A sling may help immobilize a fractured arm. An open fracture can get infected, so cover the wound with sterile gauze before applying a splint.

If the person appears faint or pale, or is breathing in a shallow, rapid fashion, treat the person for shock (see page 200). Lay the person down, elevate the legs, and cover him or her with a blanket to keep warm. Lay the person on the uninjured side if vomiting occurs.

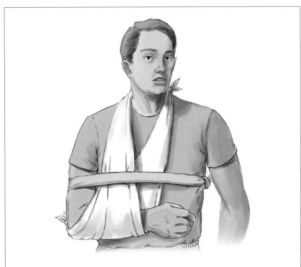

A simple sling can effectively immobilize an injured elbow.

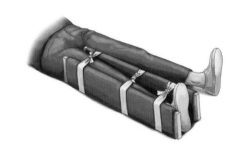

A splint can be made of wood, metal or any rigid material. Pad the splint with gauze or cloth, and then fasten the splint to the limb with gauze or strips of cloth, tape or other material.

Heart attack

Some heart attacks occur suddenly, but most start slowly, with mild pain or discomfort. The symptoms may come and go, over minutes or over hours.

If you suspect you're having a heart attack, call 911 or emergency medical help immediately. Most people wait several hours before seeking assistance — either because they don't recognize the signs and symptoms or because they deny something could be wrong.

Each year, more than a million Americans have heart attacks — and many die because of delayed treatment. Among those who survive, most permanent damage to the heart happens in the first few hours after onset.

Minutes matter

A heart attack occurs when an artery that supplies oxygen to your heart muscle becomes blocked. Arterial blockage is often caused by a buildup of fatty deposits called plaques. Without oxygen, heart cells are destroyed, causing pain or pressure. With each passing minute, more of the heart muscle is deprived of oxygen and deteriorates or dies.

Signs and symptoms

About half the people who have heart attacks experience warning signs hours, days or even weeks in advance. Not all of the signs and symptoms listed here will occur, but the more of them you have, the more likely it's a heart attack.
- Pain, pressure, tightness, squeezing or burning in the chest lasting more than a few minutes (the sensation may come and go, triggered by exertion and relieved by rest)
- Pain in one or both arms, neck or jaw, or between the shoulder blades (with or without chest pain)*

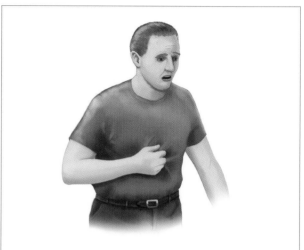

The symptoms of a heart attack vary, but you may experience pain, pressure or a squeezing sensation in your chest along with sweating and shortness of breath.

- Shortness of breath (with or without chest pain)*†
- Stomach pain or discomfort*
- Nausea or vomiting*
- Rapid, fluttering or pounding heartbeats
- Lightheadedness or dizziness
- Sweating
- Unusual fatigue for no apparent reason
- Anxiety or sense of doom

Signs and symptoms of heart attack vary widely and may differ between sexes. Some people, especially those with diabetes, have "silent" heart attacks — mild symptoms or none at all.

These symptoms are slightly more common in women than in men. Most women have some form of chest discomfort with a heart attack, but it might not be the main symptom.

† Shortness of breath without chest pain is a more common symptom of heart attack in people over age 65 and in people with diabetes.

Heart attack

Get help fast

Don't wait if you suspect a heart attack. Immediately call 911 or emergency medical help. Paramedics can treat you on the way to the hospital. If you can't access an emergency number, have someone drive you to the nearest hospital. Driving yourself can put others at risk.

While waiting for help

- Chew aspirin, if recommended by the paramedic — either one regular-strength (325 mg) tablet or four baby (81 mg each) tablets. This may help reduce the damage to your heart by making your blood less likely to clot. Chew even if you're on daily aspirin therapy because chewing (versus swallowing) speeds absorption. Don't follow this step if you're allergic to aspirin, or you have bleeding problems, or your doctor previously told you not to take aspirin.
- Take nitroglycerin, if prescribed. Using this medication according to instructions can temporarily open your blood vessels and improve blood flow to your heart. Never take anyone else's nitroglycerin medication.

When providing assistance

If you're helping someone while waiting for paramedics to arrive:
- Have the person chew aspirin as described in the section above.
- If the person becomes unconscious, begin CPR (see pages 189-191). If you're not fully trained in the procedure, you can do hands-only CPR. Most emergency medical dispatchers can instruct you in how to proceed with CPR until help arrives.

- In the initial minutes, a heart attack can trigger ventricular fibrillation, a condition in which the heart quivers uselessly. Without immediate attention, ventricular fibrillation leads to sudden death. The timely use of an automated external defibrillator (AED) — which helps shock the heart back into a normal rhythm — can provide emergency assistance before the person having a heart attack reaches a hospital. For more on AEDs, see page 189.

Prevention

A healthy lifestyle can help you prevent a heart attack by controlling risk factors that contribute to the narrowing of the arteries that supply blood to your heart. Aspects of a healthy lifestyle include:
- Not smoking and avoiding secondhand smoke
- Staying physically active
- Eating a heart-healthy diet
- Maintaining a healthy weight
- Managing stress
- Getting regular medical checkups
- Controlling blood pressure and cholesterol

You may also be advised to take a daily aspirin.

Poisoning

Any substance swallowed, inhaled, injected or absorbed by the body that interferes with the body's normal function can be, by definition, a poison.

Pesticides and household cleaning supplies are well-known poisons, but there are many other less familiar substances that may poison you. In fact, almost any nonfood substance is poisonous if taken in large enough doses.

Signs and symptoms

Poisoning can be a serious medical emergency. Look for these warning signs if you suspect poisoning has occurred:
- Unconsciousness
- Burns or redness around the mouth and lips
- Breath that smells like chemicals or gasoline
- Vomiting, difficulty breathing, drowsiness or confusion
- Uncontrollable restlessness or agitation or having seizures
- Burns, stains and odors on the person, on clothing, or on the furniture, rugs or other objects in the surrounding area
- Empty medication bottles or scattered pills

What you can do

If someone is unconscious and you think that he or she has ingested poison, call immediately for emergency medical help.

If the person is awake and alert, take the following steps:
- If the person has been exposed to poisonous fumes, such as carbon monoxide, get him or her into fresh air immediately. Avoid breathing in the fumes yourself.
- Call Poison Help at 800-222-1222 in the United States.
- When you call for emergency assistance, have the following information ready, if possible:
  - The person's condition, age and weight.
  - The ingredients listed on the product container, if available.
  - The approximate time that the poisoning took place.
  - Your name, phone number and location.
- Follow the directions provided by Poison Help for treatment.
- Don't allow the person to eat or drink anything unless instructed to do so. Don't administer ipecac syrup to induce vomiting.
- Monitor vital signs and changes in the person. who was poisoned. If breathing stops, begin CPR (see pages 189-192). Watch for symptoms of shock (see page 200).
- If poison has spilled on the person's clothing, skin or eyes, remove the clothing, using gloves. Rinse the skin in a shower or flush the eyes with water.
- Take the poison container or packaging with you to the hospital, if available.

Caution with kids

Children under age 5 are often exposed to poisons because they're curious and they're unaware of the danger. If infants and toddlers live in or visit your home:
- Keep potential poisons in cabinets located out of reach, or with safety locks.
- Keep the Poison Help phone number handy: 800-222-1222.

Seizure

A seizure occurs when sudden, abnormal brain cell activity affects the way your brain coordinates information. A seizure can produce temporary confusion, uncontrollable jerking movements and complete loss of consciousness. Some seizures are more severe than others. However, all seizures should be treated as medical emergencies.

Seizures caused by epilepsy are perhaps the best known kind, but several other disorders can produce them, including head injury, heart rhythm problem and sudden withdrawal from certain medications.

People with diabetes may experience insulin shock, which may produce a form of seizure that is treated differently than other seizures.

What you can do

When you're with a person who is having a seizure:

1. Keep the person from injuring himself or herself. If vomiting occurs, turn the person's head so that the vomit is expelled and isn't breathed in. Clear the area around the person of furniture or other objects to reduce his or her risk of injury during uncontrolled body movements. Although the person may briefly stop breathing, breathing almost invariably returns without need for CPR.
2. After the seizure is over, position the person on his or her side to allow for normal breathing and for vomit, blood and other fluids to drain from the mouth. Blood may be present if he or she bit the tongue or cheek. The person may be confused for a while. Monitor changes until there's a complete return of mental function.
3. Seek emergency assistance during a seizure if necessary. Call for immediate help if:
   - The person has never had a seizure before
   - The episode lasts more than a few minutes
   - The seizure reoccurs

4. Treat any bumps, bruises or cuts that may have occurred during the seizure, particularly if there was a fall.

Insulin shock

A person with diabetes may experience a seizure if his or her blood sugar drops too low. This form of seizure is called insulin shock.

If you're with someone experiencing insulin shock, give the person some kind of carbohydrate or sugar, if possible. Fruit juices, candy or sugar-containing soft drinks are effective.

If the person is unable to swallow, try putting a teaspoon of syrup in his or her cheek every few minutes. If the person is unconscious, you may need to administer a glucagon injection under the skin using a special injector. If recovery isn't prompt, seek immediate medical attention.

Seizure in a child

Sometimes, a high fever in an infant or child can cause what's known as a febrile seizure. If this situation occurs, stay calm and follow these steps:

- Place your child on his or her side, at a location where there's no chance of falling.
- Stay close to watch and comfort your child.
- Remove any hard or sharp objects near your child.
- Loosen any tight or restrictive clothing.
- Don't restrain your child or interfere with your child's movements.
- Don't attempt to put anything in your child's mouth.

A first-time seizure should be evaluated by your doctor as soon as possible, even if it lasts only a few seconds. If the seizure lasts longer than five minutes or is accompanied by vomiting, stiff neck, breathing difficulty or extreme sleepiness, seek emergency medical attention.

Shock

Shock may result from trauma, heatstroke, allergic reaction, severe infection, poisoning, dehydration or other causes. When you're in shock, there's a reduction of blood flow throughout your body — a change that lowers your blood pressure and reduces the supply of oxygen to organs and other vital tissues. Shock can come on suddenly or it can have a delayed onset. The condition can be life-threatening.

Signs and symptoms

Various signs and symptoms may appear when a person is in shock:

- Change in skin color and feel. The skin may look pale or gray, and feel cool and clammy.
- The pulse may be weak and rapid as blood pressure drops. Breathing may be slow and shallow, or rapid and deep (hyperventilation).
- The eyes lack luster and seem to stare. Sometimes the pupils are dilated.
- The person may become unconscious. If not, the person may feel faint, dizzy or weak, or become confused, or extremely anxious or agitated.

What you can do

If you suspect that a person is going into shock, even if there were no warning signs immediately after an injury, call 911 or emergency medical help. There may be a delayed reaction. While waiting for emergency responders to arrive:

1. Lay the person down on his or her back with a cushion or other prop elevating the feet higher than the head. If raising the legs will cause pain or further injury, keep the body flat. Keep movement to a minimum.
2. Keep the person warm and comfortable. Loosen tight collars, belts and clothing that constricts. Cover the person with a blanket. If the ground or floor is cold, place a blanket underneath. If it's hot, place the person in the shade or a cool area, if possible. Even if the person complains of thirst, give nothing to drink.
3. Watch for warning signs of shock. Check for breathing and a pulse. If the signs are absent, begin CPR (see pages 189-192).
4. If the person vomits or bleeds from the mouth, turn the person on his or her side to prevent choking.
5. Start treatment for bleeding or injuries, such as broken bones, if you can. Immobilize a fracture or take other first-aid steps.

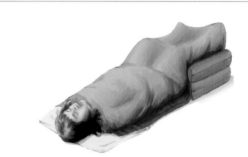

With the onset of shock, keep the person warm, and elevate legs and feet above the level of the heart in order to maximize the flow of blood to the head.

Stroke

In the United States, stroke is the fifth-leading cause of death, resulting in one out of every 20 deaths. It's also a leading cause of adult disability.

A stroke is a "brain attack" — it happens when blood supply to a part of your brain is interrupted or severely reduced. Within a few minutes of being deprived of oxygen and nutrients, brain cells in that area begin dying.

A stroke is a medical emergency, and prompt treatment is crucial. Almost 2 million brain cells die each minute during a typical stroke. As the American Heart Association notes, "With a stroke, time lost is brain lost."

Signs and symptoms

To help you recognize a stroke, think "FAST:"
- Face. Ask the person to smile. Does one side of the face droop?
- Arms. Ask the person to raise both arms. Does one arm drift downward? Or is the person unable to lift one arm?
- Speech. Ask the person to repeat a simple phrase. Is his or her speech slurred or strange?
- Time. If you observe any of these signs, call 911 or emergency medical help immediately.

Signs and symptoms may last only minutes, or they may persist for hours. Warning signs should be taken very seriously.

What you can do

If you suspect that you're experiencing warning signs of stroke, call 911 or emergency medical help immediately.

If you're calling for another person, monitor him or her closely while waiting for the emergency responders. Be ready to take these actions, if necessary:
- If breathing stops, begin CPR (see pages 189-191). Minor breathing difficulty may be relieved simply by resting the person's head and shoulders on a pillow.
- If vomiting occurs, turn the person's head to the side so that the vomit can drain out of the mouth instead of into the lungs. Don't allow the person to eat or drink anything.
- If paralysis occurs, protect the paralyzed limbs from injury that might occur when the person moves about or is transported.

What's a TIA?

A transient ischemic attack (TIA) has the similar signs and symptoms of a stroke but usually lasts only a few minutes and causes no permanent damage. Often called a ministroke, a TIA can serve as a warning — each TIA attack increases your risk of a stroke.

If you think you've had a TIA, call your doctor immediately. After a TIA, your risk of a stroke increases immediately and may be as high as 10 to 20 percent over the next three months. The doctor may identify potentially treatable conditions that may help you prevent a future stroke — for example, high blood pressure, high cholesterol or diabetes. The doctor may also prescribe medication to prevent blood clots or a procedure to remove the buildup of plaques in your arteries.

Index

W

warts, 180

watery eyes, 181

weight loss
    arthritis and, 16
    asthma and, 18
    chronic pain and, 39
    diabetes and, 57
    high cholesterol and, 103
    snoring and, 152, 153

wrinkles, 182

wrist and hand pain, 183

Y

yoga
    for arthritis, 16
    for back pain, 21
    for chronic pain, 40
    for stress and anxiety, 162

Z

zinc, 44

MAYO CLINIC
Housecall

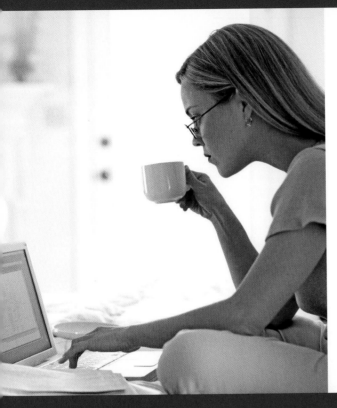

What our readers are saying ...

*"I depend on **Mayo Clinic Housecall** more than any other medical info that shows up on my computer. Thank you so very much."*

"Excellent newsletter. I always find something interesting to read and learn something new."

*"**Housecall** is a must read – keep up the good work!"*

*"I love **Housecall**. It is one of the most useful, trusted and beneficial things that come from the Internet."*

*"The **Housecall** is timely, interesting and invaluable in its information. Thanks much to Mayo Clinic for this resource!"*

"I enjoy getting the weekly newsletters. They provide me with friendly reminders, as well as information/ conditions I was not aware of."

Get the latest health information direct from Mayo Clinic ... Sign up today, it's FREE!

Mayo Clinic Housecall is a FREE weekly e-newsletter that offers the latest health information from the experts at Mayo Clinic. Stay up to date on topics that are current, interesting, and most of all important to your health and the health of your family.

What you get
- Weekly top story
- Additional healthy highlights
- Answers from the experts
- Quick access to trusted health tools
- Featured blogs
- Health tip of the week
- Special offers

Don't wait ... Join today!
MayoClinic.com/Housecall/Register

We're committed to helping you enjoy better health and get the most out of life every day. We hope you decide to become part of the Mayo Clinic family, where you can always count on receiving an interesting mix of health information from a trusted source.

Experts. Answers.
Mayo Clinic.

For complex medical conditions, answers can be hard to find. At Mayo Clinic, world-class experts work together, across specialties, to make sure you get exactly the care you need—care that's also covered by most insurance plans. It's a seamless approach to delivering complex care.

Make your appointment at **mayoclinic.org**.

MAYO
CLINIC